AFRICAN ISSUES

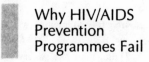

# 'Letting Them Die'

## Why HIV/AIDS Prevention Programmes Fail

*'In the old South Africa we killed people.*

*Now we're just letting them die.'*

Pieter-Dirk Uys, South African satirist

## AFRICAN ISSUES

Published in the US & Canada by Indiana University Press

**Undermining Development** The Absence of Power among Local NGOS in Africa
SARAH MICHAEL

**'Letting them Die'** Why HIV/AIDS Prevention Programmes Fail
CATHERINE CAMPBELL

**Somalia: Economy without State** Accumulation & Survival in Somalia
PETER D. LITTLE

**The Root Causes of Sudan's Civil Wars**
DOUGLAS H. JOHNSON

**Asbestos Blues** Labour, Capital, Physicians & the State in South Africa
JOCK McCULLOCH

**Fortress Conservation** The Preservation of the Mkomazi Game Reserve, Tanzania
DAN BROCKINGTON

**Killing for Conservation** Wildlife Policy in Zimbabwe
ROSALEEN DUFFY

**Mozambique & the Great Flood of 2000**
FRANCES CHRISTIE & JOSEPH HANLON

**Angola: Anatomy of an Oil State**
TONY HODGES

**Congo-Paris** Transnational Traders on the Margins of the Law
JANET MACGAFFEY & REMY BAZENGUISSA-GANGA

**Africa Works** Disorder as Political Instrument
PATRICK CHABAL & JEAN-PASCAL DALOZ

**The Criminalization of the State in Africa**
JEAN-FRANÇOIS BAYART, STEPHEN ELLIS & BEATRICE HIBOU

**Famine Crimes** Politics & the Disaster Relief Industry in Africa
ALEX DE WAAL

Published in the US & Canada by Heinemann (N.H.)

**Peace without Profit** How the IMF Blocks Rebuilding in Mozambique
JOSEPH HANLON

**The Lie of the Land** Challenging the Received Wisdom on the African Environment
MELISSA LEACH & ROBIN MEARNS (eds)

**Fighting for the Rainforest** War, Youth & Resources in Sierra Leone
PAUL RICHARDS

AFRICAN ISSUES

# 'Letting Them Die'

## Why HIV/AIDS Prevention Programmes Fail

CATHERINE CAMPBELL

Department of Social Psychology
London School of Economics
& Political Science

The International
African Institute

*in association with*

JAMES CURREY
Oxford

INDIANA UNIVERSITY PRESS
Bloomington & Indianapolis

DOUBLE STOREY/a Juta company
Cape Town

The International    James Currey
African Institute    73 Botley Road
in association with    Oxford OX2 0BS

Double Storey Books,    Indiana University Press
a Juta company    601 North Morton Street
Mercury Crescent    Bloomington
Wetton 7780    Indiana 47404
(North America)

**British Library Cataloguing in Publication Data**

Campbell, Catherine
'Letting them die' : why HIV/AIDS intervention programmes
fail. – (African issues)
1.AIDS (Disease) – South Africa 2.AIDS (Diseases – South
Africa – Prevention
I.Title
362.1'969792'00968

ISBN 10: 0-85255-868-6 (James Currey paper)
ISBN 13: 978-0 85255-868-3 (James Currey paper)

**Library of Congress Cataloging-in-Publication Data**

A catalog record for this book is available from the Library of Congress

ISBN 10: 0-253-21635-4 (Indiana paper)
ISBN 13: 978-0-253-21635-9 (Indiana paper)

*Typeset by*
Saxon Graphics Ltd, Derby
in 9/11 Melior with Optima display

Printed and bound in Great Britain
by Woolnough, Irthlingborough

# CONTENTS

# ACKNOWLEDGEMENTS

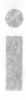

This book is the result of seven years of collaborative research and thinking, and my debt to colleagues is understandably a large one. My greatest debt is to Brian Williams, instigator and driving force behind the research. Brian set up the Summertown HIV-Prevention Project, and co-ordinated it for the three-year period under scrutiny in this book, as well as serving as Principal Investigator on the Project. This book was enabled by his deep commitment to the development of social understandings of the HIV/AIDS epidemic, in addition to biomedical and epidemiological ones. His passion, enthusiasm and creativity created a unique opportunity for social research and reflection in a biomedically dominated research arena. Working in his research team was a great privilege – if somewhat hectic at times. Brian was co-author of a number of papers on which I drew in putting this book together.

Catherine MacPhail played the central role in the data collection and research management. Catherine has been a highly valued friend, colleague and sounding board over a four-year period. This book would not have been possible without her hard work, support and determination to conduct rigorous research under challenging circumstances. It is Catherine's personal research into sexuality and HIV-prevention among young people that forms the basis of Chapters 7 and 8 of this book. She was also a co-author of unpublished research reports that I drew on in writing Chapters 2, 6, 9 and 10.

It was Zodwa Mzaidume, the Community Outreach Co-ordinator of the Summertown Project, who co-ordinated the sex worker peer education programme that forms the subject of Chapters 4, 5 and 6. The research reported on here is deeply marked by Zodwa's inspirational community mobilization skills, her in-depth understanding of community dynamics and her generosity in sharing her experiences through her participation in the process evaluation of the Summertown Project peer education programme. This book bears many traces of her generosity and patience in being prepared to engage in the often-fraught process of engagement between activists and academics.

Having acknowledged my deep indebtedness to these three colleagues, I must emphasize that I take full personal responsibility for the ideas expressed in this book. While colleagues helped me with the content of particular chapters, the analytical framework is the result of my own work, and the conclusions and arguments of the book do not in any way intend to reflect the views and opinions of my colleagues.

The bulk of this research was funded by the British Department for International Development (DfID). (In the final stages of the research small contributions were received from the US Population Council Horizons Project and UN AIDS.) Here again I must emphasize that while I am indebted to these agencies for their generosity, the ideas in this book are my own, and do not represent the views of the research funders.

I am grateful to *Social Science and Medicine* for permission to reproduce material from Campbell (1997),[1] Campbell (2000),[2] MacPhail and Campbell (2001)[3] and Campbell and MacPhail (2002).[4] Thanks also to the *American Journal of Public Health* for permission to reproduce material from Campbell and Mzaidume (2001),[5] and to the *Journal of Community and Applied Social Psychology* for material from Campbell and Jovchelovitch (2000).[6]

Particular thanks are due to all the members of the Summertown community who agreed to participate in our research interviews and focus groups. I thank them for their patience and support. Solly Moema manages the Summertown Project Implementation Team, and Bareng Rasego is the Clinical Services Co-ordinator. They have played a key role in making this research possible. Thanks to them for their support and insights, offered in detailed discussions of this material at various stages of the research. Thanks also to Lewis Ndhlovu, David Wilson, Bertran Auvert, Dirk Taljaard, Julian Lambert, Tony Davies and David Ginsburg for useful discussions at various stages of the work. Cheeks Macheke was co-author of a paper that I draw on in Chapter 1, and Roy Williams authored a report that I draw on in Chapters 9 and 10.

Large numbers of people have assisted at various stages of the knowledge production process. There are too many to mention by name, but they include: Cheeks Macheke, Oupa Raymond Matsi, Khosi Mashiyane, Theodora Sogiba, Colleen Summerson, Jeannette de Bruyn, Tshetlha Phuteho, Jeannette Lesoetsa, Caroline Nohamatu, Rethabile Nkopane, Nonkululeko Mnunu, Ephraim Sikhuza, Gaph Phatedi, Ausi Mohlambane, Phampang Manato, Sello Molefe, Mampine Macheka, Claudia Mbatha, Brenda Mashlambi, Lerato Goge, Lesego Shika, Prudence and Essie Ngoako, David Molebatsi, Phyllis Serobatse, Palesa Nxumalo, Mamokete Ramasike and Mr Babophe.

My ability to conduct this work has been heavily dependent on the goodwill and tolerance of colleagues in the Social Psychology Department at the London School of Economics (LSE), who made space for my frequent trips to South Africa. In particular, I continue to benefit from my ongoing collaboration with Sandra Jovchelovitch, co-author of a paper that I draw on extensively in Chapter 3; Steve Bennett, who provided various invaluable forms of technical assistance; and Carl

McLean, who assisted extensively with the collection of background material. I have also benefited from intellectual discussions with Tony Klouda, Fiona Meth, Paula Meth, Charles Meth, Hélène Joffe, Grahame Hayes and Pamela Gillies. Detailed comments on the manuscript were kindly given by Mike Kirkwood, Simon Gregson, Urban Jonsson, Joy de Beyer, David Simon, Jo Beall, Teddy Brett, Brian Williams, Alex de Waal and Roy Williams. Their critical insights and suggestions have greatly improved the final product, though here again I must emphasize that colleagues did not always agree with all the views expressed in the pages that follow. Particular thanks to Alex de Waal for enabling me to publish this book in the African Issues series. At the personal level I have relied heavily on the support of Martyn Corbett and Sheila Newman. Last, but not least, particular thanks to my partner Harry Grusin for support and encouragement way beyond the call of duty.

*Catherine Campbell*
*Social Psychology, London School of Economics*

# INTRODUCTION

## Sexuality, Participation & Social Change

Why is it that people knowingly engage in sexual behaviour that could lead to a slow and painful premature death? Why do the best-intentioned attempts to stem the tide of the HIV epidemic often have so little impact? In answering these questions attention will be given to the phenomenon of sexuality, and the way it is shaped and constrained by factors ranging from the deepest psychological needs for intimacy and pleasure, to the complex and unequal relationships between women and men, rich and poor, and between North and South. In particular, attention will be given to the social construction of sexuality by migrant mineworkers, commercial sex workers and young people in the small South African community of Summertown,[1] all of whom, albeit in different ways, live in situations that place them at particularly high risk of HIV infection.

In addition to this focus on the construction of sexuality, this book also examines some of the obstacles and challenges facing HIV-prevention programmes. It does so through a detailed study of the Summertown Project, a project that worked to limit the spread of HIV among these three groups. Like most development projects, this one used the methods of 'community participation' and 'multi-stakeholder partnerships' to address its goals. In particular it sought to promote two forms of participation and partnership. Firstly, it sought to promote a series of community-led peer education programmes within a variety of Summertown groups that were at particularly high risk of HIV infection. Secondly, it sought to promote partnerships or alliances between a diverse array of community groupings and relevant agencies from the private and public sectors and civil society ('stakeholders') – in the interests of co-ordinating and supporting the variety of local HIV-prevention efforts in such a way that maximized their overall cumulative effectiveness. The concepts of participation and partnerships serve as articles of faith in development projects around the world. Yet understanding of the processes whereby participation or partnerships might achieve their allegedly beneficial effects is still in its infancy. A central goal of this book is to understand how and why participation might lead to improved sexual health, as well as to highlight the possibilities and limitations of local participation as a method for changing the contexts of sexuality within which the HIV epidemic flourishes.

The Summertown Project sought to mobilize the local mining community to address a problem that threatens to kill up to six out of ten of its young women, and four out of ten of its young men. These will be young people in the prime of their economic and reproductive lives, and HIV/AIDS will kill them before they have brought up their children, cared for their elderly parents or made their contribution to the economy. Why so many deaths? They are not due to ignorance. Most people in Summertown have a good grasp of the facts about HIV – that it is sexually transmitted, that there is currently no cure, and that its spread can be prevented by the use of condoms. This book will seek to answer this question by telling the interlinked stories of four groups of people: miners, sex workers, young people and the group loosely referred to as Summertown's 'stakeholders' (representatives of a diverse array of groupings – but all with an interest in the health and well-being of people in Summertown). Each of these stories contributes one piece to the complex puzzle of why it is that people continue to knowingly dice with death by taking sexual health risks, and why it is so difficult to alter this situation.

## Community level of analysis

The task of understanding the transmission and prevention of HIV/AIDS is one that involves attention to a range of academic disciplines and levels of analysis. At the outset it must be emphasized that this book has a very specific focus. The author is a social psychologist, with a particular interest in the local community level of analysis.[2] To date this level of analysis has been relatively neglected in HIV science. At the micro-social level, HIV/AIDS has already been well covered by health psychologists, who have been strongly represented in the academic study of sexual behaviour. They have produced a steady stream of scholarly studies, linking sexual behaviour to properties of the individual, such as cognitive processes, instincts, attitudes, sense of personal vulnerability, or perceived social norms. At the macro-social level, economists, anthropologists and sociologists have drawn attention to the way in which factors such as poverty, gender inequalities and global capitalism shape the contexts within which the epidemic flourishes. Each of these perspectives forms an essential frame in the kaleidoscope of factors that are implicated in the development and persistence of the HIV epidemic in developing countries, making a crucial contribution to understandings in this area.[3] However, less attention has been paid to the way in which these micro and macro factors interact at the local community level.

The community level of analysis is important for two reasons. Firstly, communities serve as key mediators between the macro- and micro-social levels of analysis mentioned above. Local communities often form the contexts within which people negotiate their social and sexual lives and identities. As will be illustrated in this book, they equally often play a key role in enabling or restraining people from taking control over their health. In playing this enabling or restraining role, communities are profoundly structured by the broader economic and gendered relations of the wider societies in which they are located, and deeply implicated in the processes whereby factors such as poverty and gender inequalities translate themselves into the most intimate areas of people's lives.

Secondly, there is now widespread agreement that a key step in addressing the HIV epidemic is to get local people collectively to 'take ownership' of the problem, engaging in collective action to increase the likelihood that people will act in health-enhancing ways, and to mobilize for the creation of community contexts that enable improved sexual health. In the light of the limited successes of biomedical and behavioural approaches in achieving large-scale reductions in HIV, a growing range of voices are pointing to the potential contribution of community-level approaches to bringing about such changes in the 'hard-to-reach' communities that are often the most vulnerable to HIV infection.

A key aim of this book's focus on the psycho-social and community-level determinants of sexuality is to highlight the importance of – and the immense complexities of – mobilizing a wide variety of stakeholder groups in developing new health and social systems that might contribute to addressing the complexity of the HIV/AIDS phenomenon. In Summertown, these local groups include, for example, destitute sex workers eking out a living in conditions of poverty and violence, local township groupings representing constituencies such as women or young people or churches, well-heeled representatives of the powerful mining industry, government health departments, and overseas donor agencies charged with promoting 'development in Africa'. This book will also highlight the need for new conceptual frameworks for understanding health and sexuality, and for informing intervention and policy in the field of sexual health. Change and innovation are of particular importance in relation to an epidemic such as HIV because epidemics are, by definition, extraordinary events. They arise because existing understandings of health and illness, and existing public health systems and institutions, are inappropriate for addressing the particular form the epidemic takes, and for stemming the particular mechanisms by which it spreads.[4] The possibility of universally accessible and totally effective treatments or cures for HIV/AIDS remains remote in the less advantaged countries and contexts where the epidemic often has its strongest hold. Within such a context, the challenge of containing it requires innovation and change in relation to both frameworks of understanding and modes of action and intervention.

The dangers of the epidemic are now unavoidably clear. There is also a growing awareness that the suffering and damage already sustained are only minor compared to the devastation that could lie ahead if nothing is done.[5] Furthermore, there is now evidence that through a combination of well-co-ordinated 'top-down' and 'bottom-up' action some less affluent countries have managed to lower infection rates and to lessen the suffering of those affected by the epidemic.[6] Yet, despite this, a range of barriers stands in the way of the development of new modes of understanding, action and intervention in other countries. This book seeks to highlight such barriers and constraints, in the interests of marking out the challenges that lie ahead.

## Reaffirming a commitment to HIV-prevention

HIV/AIDS has caused indescribable suffering to millions of people. In 2002 alone, 5 million people were infected, bringing the global total of people were living with HIV/AIDS to 42 million. While it has become common to refer to it as an epidemic of globalization, and while much publicity has been given to its impact on people in the wealthy countries of North America and Western Europe, its effects are concentrated very heavily in the less affluent areas of the world. Thus, for example, while North America has 980 000 people living with HIV/AIDS, Western Europe 570 000, and Australia and New Zealand 15 000, UN AIDS[7] figures suggest that 29.4 million people are affected in sub-Saharan Africa, where more than 11 million children have been orphaned by AIDS. Furthermore, while figures in Eastern Europe and Asia are currently relatively low compared to Africa, standing at 1 200 000 in Eastern Europe and Central Asia, and 6 000 000 in South and South East Asia, a dramatic increase is predicted in countries such as India, China, the Ukraine and Russia over the next twenty years.

HIV/AIDS threatens to wipe out decades of development gains in the world's poorer countries, as measured by life expectancy. Average life expectancy in sub-Saharan Africa – which would have been 62 years without AIDS – is now 47 years. In Botswana, it has dropped to 36, a level last seen in 1950. In Lesotho, a person who turned 15 in 2000 has a 74 per cent chance of becoming infected before his or her fiftieth birthday. AIDS' negative impact on life expectancy is also felt beyond Africa, albeit less dramatically. Haiti's life expectancy is nearly six years less than it would have been without AIDS, and in Cambodia it is four years less. In Guyana, the probability of becoming HIV-positive between the ages of 15 and 50 is 19 per cent.[8]

HIV/AIDS is a disease that ravages every aspect of people's lives, from the most intimate to the most public. Intricately entangled with the taboo topics of sex and death, it is a disease that has repeatedly captured the public imagination, as well as an unprecedented amount of public attention and money. The UN Security Council has called it an international security issue. Billions of dollars are being allocated to fighting the disease,[9] and it is rapidly becoming one of the best-researched diseases in human history. Yet while a handful of countries seem to have contained its spread to a greater or lesser extent, in other contexts HIV/AIDS continues its relentless march from one country to another.

The sheer scale of the devastation left in its wake commands attention, with hundreds of thousands of people infected worldwide every day. The enormity of these impersonal statistics often masks the depth and scope of the personal pain and suffering associated with each individual case. The disease targets people in the prime of their economic and child-rearing lives. It ravages the life chances of children, some before they are even born, with high rates of mother-to-child transmission of the disease. It also has the power to devastate the lives of those children who are HIV-free. It creates households headed by children as young as nine years old acting as guardians to younger siblings, sometimes with no source of income. Having weathered the trauma of losing parents the high rates of mother-to-child transmission means that these children will now have to care for terminally ill younger siblings.

The experience of very many people living with HIV/AIDS in southern Africa appears to be one of deepening poverty, isolation and an inability to satisfy basic needs such as food and shelter. Given the stigma and terror that surrounds the disease in the public imagination, people live in fear of rejection by their communities and formal health services, and fear for their children. Because of a fear of rejection, people living with HIV/AIDS are often reluctant to seek out or access services, opting instead to live without support or treatment. Those who disclose their status often become victims of violence, either from partners or family members, or from communities where HIV is regarded with fear, denial and stigma.

The fight against HIV/AIDS is one of the biggest challenges facing sub-Saharan Africa over the next decade, and the impact of the disease will touch on the lives of the global community in myriad predictable and unpredictable ways. Despite the enormity of the crisis, biomedical and pharmaceutical developments and responses have been slow to develop. Attempts to develop vaccines continue to have limited success. The amount spent on researching AIDS vaccines remains relatively little (between $300 million and $600 million dollars a year) and focuses predominantly on strains of HIV found mainly in the US and Western Europe.[10] While there has been more success in the development of anti-retroviral drugs, which are prolonging thousands of lives in wealthy countries, as well as among the wealthy minority in the less affluent world, these drugs continue to remain inaccessible to the bulk of those affected. Thus, for example, at the end of 2001 it was estimated that only 30 000 of the 28.5 million people living with HIV/AIDS in sub-Saharan Africa had access to antiretroviral drugs.[11] In short, there is little hope of pharmaceutical solutions being available in ways that can be affordably and effectively implemented in the short-term future by many of the poorest countries where HIV flourishes. Prevention, through encouraging safer sexual behaviour, remains a key weapon against HIV.

Ongoing attention to international debates and struggles about making drug treatment available to poorer countries is clearly vitally important. The intensity of the suffering endured by people living with AIDS and their families cannot be underestimated. Furthermore, the provision of humane and effective treatment is part and parcel of the HIV-prevention struggle, given that people are most likely to be open about their fears of infection, seek out information about prevention, and present themselves for voluntary counselling and testing in conditions where they see that AIDS-sufferers are treated with dignity and respect, and where real help is available to those who ascertain and disclose their HIV status. However, debate and activism regarding treatment must not be allowed to create a false sense of complacency about the continued dangers of infection, or to divert attention away from the importance of ongoing prevention efforts. It is not entirely clear whether even the best treatment strategies will be able to contain the virus for an extended period in the majority of HIV-infected individuals, or lead to total eradication of the virus. Treatments are expensive, have negative side effects, are difficult to administer in deprived settings, and difficult to stick to for long periods.

Even if and when money becomes available to buy HIV/AIDS drugs for all those who need them, much work will remain to be done in achieving the sustainable development of health systems capable of successfully implementing complex treatment regimes. In South Africa particular provinces and cities have relatively advanced health care facilities. Others, however, lack the physical, human and organizational infrastructure to implement even the relatively simple six-month drug treatments for tuberculosis, or the basic immunization of children, let alone the far more complex long-term demands of administering complex AIDS drugs.[12] In 1998 only 63.4 per cent of South African children were immunized, with full immunization coverage in two provinces as low as 49.5 per cent and 52.6 per cent, for example.[13] In some provinces as few as 10 per cent of tuberculosis patients adhere to the much simpler treatments than HIV/AIDS drugs, which only have to be taken for six months.[14]

Even when drugs are readily available and where there are systems in place for ensuring that people take them properly, the possibility of drug resistance poses problems. Drug-resistant HIV has a relatively high prevalence. It can be transmitted from an infected person to an uninfected person; it can 'super-infect' people who are already HIV-positive; and it may even increase HIV incidence among at-risk populations.

Against this background it is sometimes alarming to see how the issue of drugs often has the potential to draw energy and attention away from debates about prevention. There is an urgent need for academics, activists and health workers to reaffirm their commitment to recognition of the importance of HIV/AIDS prevention in curbing the epidemic.

## Poor understandings of sexuality

Many existing HIV-prevention efforts in sub-Saharan Africa have been dominated by the very biomedical and behavioural understandings of sexuality and health that allowed the epidemic to develop in the first place. If prevention efforts are to have optimal impact they need to be informed by sound insights into the determinants of sex and sexuality. Yet these are arguably the most mysterious and multi-faceted aspects of human behaviour. Early in the HIV epidemic, it was often assumed that sexual behaviour was shaped by the conscious decisions of rational individuals. Locating the cause of sexual behaviour at the individual level led to individual behavioural interventions. Optimistic sexual health promoters assumed that if only one could reach HIV-vulnerable people and tell them about the dangers of HIV and how to prevent it, they would quickly take care to safeguard their behaviour. 'It's as easy as A, B, C (Abstain, Be faithful or Condomize)' became a familiar slogan in many African countries. When research showed that having other sexually transmitted infections (STIs) increased one's chance of getting HIV, health promoters worked to step up STI treatment services in the same vein.

But one study after another – as well as rocketing AIDS statistics – have shown that people often knowingly engage in sexual behaviour that places their health at risk. With full knowledge of the dangers of the epidemic, many people continue to have unprotected sex, often with multiple partners. Furthermore, while well-funded research studies conducted in carefully managed settings have shown that treating STIs reduces HIV prevalence, in real-life situations out of the context of such well-resourced and carefully managed studies, people often fail to present at STI treatment facilities at the first signs of infection, despite knowing that the presence of other STIs increases their vulnerability to HIV. The forces shaping sexual behaviour and sexual health are far more complex than individual rational decisions based on simple factual knowledge about health risks, and the availability of medical services.

Other studies of sexual behaviour have sought to explain it in terms of a range of deep-seated instincts and unconscious emotions. However, more recently there has been a growing understanding that while sexuality cannot be divorced from the physical body, and from our instincts and emotions, it is also socially constructed. This has led to a series of studies that have sought to show that HIV/AIDS is in some or other way the result of 'African culture', pointing to a series of exotic tribal customs (such as scarification) that place African people at particular risk for HIV.

This book seeks to expand its gaze beyond the scope of factors such as the sexual behaviour or local culture of HIV-affected communities. It seeks to understand the transmission and prevention of HIV not as a problem 'out there in the townships' or as the product of reified exotic

African behaviours or cultural practices, but as a social issue located at the interfaces of a range of constituencies with competing actions and interests. These include not only those local communities, organizations and individuals directly affected by the epidemic, but also local and national political leaders and business groups, overseas experts and international development and funding agencies. It is hoped that such an analysis will bring about a greater understanding of the challenges facing even the best-intentioned and technically well-informed HIV-prevention interventions and policies in the complex and multi-layered situations in which they operate.

## Why such a commitment to individualistic perspectives?

Why is it that people continue to prioritize individualistic biomedical and behavioural perspectives? One answer to this question lies in the dearth of actionable understandings of the ways in which community and social contexts impact on health. Epidemiologists have done a good job of making links between HIV and quantifiable contextual variables. However, social scientists have been slow in explaining the underlying processes and mechanisms whereby contextual factors contribute to high levels of HIV-transmission. Formally, the academic field of the social science of HIV-prevention has been defined to include many other disciplines – such as economics, anthropology, politics, public health and sociology. Yet in practice psychologists, who have tended to favour individual-level conceptualizations of the causes of health behaviour, have dominated the field. Dominant among these conceptualizations are social cognition approaches, which conceptualize the individual as a rational information-processor, whose behaviour is determined by a combination of psychological factors such as individual attitudes, personal action plans and perceived social norms.[15] Social cognition models are sometimes quite successful in predicting how people behave in carefully controlled academic research studies, or in relatively affluent countries or groupings. However, there is now widespread acceptance that the potential of these models for explaining behaviours as complex as sexual behaviour, and for directing interventions in real-world settings among people in highly marginalized communities is limited.[16] Firstly, they focus almost exclusively on the proximal determinants of behaviour (such as individual behavioural intentions and perceived norms), with little attention to the way in which these proximal factors are influenced by social context. Yet, as this book will show, social context plays a key role in enabling and supporting health-enhancing behaviour change, particularly in marginalized communities in less affluent settings, where people often have even less control of their behaviour than their more privileged counterparts. Secondly, while these models have played an important role in identifying *which* individual cognitive factors are related to health-related behavioural intentions, or behaviours, they do not give much indication as to how to *change* these cognitive factors. It has recently been argued that psychologists have served to hinder HIV-prevention efforts in the developing world.[17] This is through the role that they have played in persistently directing attention towards the individual psychological aspects of sexual behaviour, and away from the social change that needs to take place to support the likelihood of healthier sexual behaviours. One of the key goals of this book is to illustrate the way in which sexual behaviour is determined by a much wider range of factors than the individual-level phenomena so dear to the hearts of psychologists.

Furthermore, the activities of research psychologists have too often been conducted within the boundaries of the academic journal and conference, far removed from cutting-edge developments in the practice of HIV-prevention. While HIV *science* is dominated by behavioural and biomedical research studies, in the past decade the *practice* of HIV-prevention has been characterized by a slow but steady 'paradigm drift'.[18] This has involved a move away from highly individual-oriented interventions, informed by narrow psychological theories, towards more participatory approaches. These practical interventions acknowledge the complex range of determinants of sexual behaviour, and emphasize the need for approaches such as community-led peer education and collaborative stakeholder partnerships that seek to promote community contexts that enable and support behaviour change. However, this move towards more community-oriented intervention techniques has not been matched by the development of understandings of the community and social changes that are often necessary preconditions for health-enhancing behaviour change. For this reason the possibility of learning lessons from successful and unsuccessful programmes is limited.

Research evaluating HIV-prevention programmes often continues to rely on quantitative survey methodologies. These include behavioural surveys that measure changes at the individual level, focusing on factors such as HIV-related knowledge or reported condom use before and after interventions have taken place. They also include biomedical surveys that measure levels of HIV and other STIs before and after the intervention. Clearly, such *outcome* measures are vital for measuring whether or not interventions have had their desired effects. However, they often contribute little to understandings of the *processes* whereby programmes do or do not succeed in having an impact on these biomedical and behavioural factors. Such approaches have little to teach us about broader determinants of programme success, such as psycho-social changes, features of the community-intervention interface and the degree of trust and identification with which members of target communities regard particular interventions, the willingness of more powerful groups to support efforts to improve health in more marginalized settings, and the role of various forms of social inequality in undermining programme efforts. They also tell us little about the extent to which the form and success of interventions is enabled or constrained by broader public health policy measures, or preconditions laid down by the overseas donors who fund a significant number of cutting-edge HIV/AIDS programmes. People running community programmes in various countries and contexts frequently repeat the same mistakes, or have to reinvent the wheel again and again owing to the lack of a conceptual framework for formulating and sharing lessons and findings from previous experiences.

Another key aim of this book is to outline such a framework for conceptualizing the processes whereby community-level interventions succeed or fail in bringing about health-enhancing behaviour change. This aim is pursued within the spirit of a critical social psychology that seeks to expand current psychological understandings of behaviour in two ways. Firstly, a critical social psychology seeks to take account of the social determinants of behaviour in addition to the individual psychological determinants. Secondly, it seeks to contribute to the development of actionable theories, in the spirit of the dictum that a social scientist's role is not just to explain behaviour, but to explain it in ways that point towards the possibility of changing it. Within the field of HIV-prevention, an 'actionable' theory is one that seeks to explain sexual behaviour in ways that have direct implications for the design of public health interventions and policies – through its attention to the complex dialectic of the individual and the community/societal levels of analysis in shaping both sexuality and the possibility of sexual behaviour change. It is this dialectic that lies at the heart of various forms of participation in collective action that have a vital role in efforts to control the HIV epidemic in marginalized communities. Ideally, such collective action provides the context within which groups of people can collaborate in efforts to change not only themselves and each other, but also to identify, and where possible to challenge, the social circumstances that have placed their health at risk.

## Health, community and participation: The role of community mobilization

Reference has already been made to the complexity of sexual behaviour, which cannot be understood simply in terms of individual decisions, or changed through giving people information. Giving people information about health risks is unlikely to change the behaviour of more than one in four people, and these are generally the more affluent and better-educated members of a social group.[1] This is because health-related behaviours (such as condom use) are determined not only by conscious rational choice by individuals, on the basis of good information, but also by the extent to which broader contextual factors support the performance of such behaviours.

This presents health promoters with the challenge of developing policies and interventions in social and community contexts that enable and support health-enhancing behaviours. However, the understanding of what constitutes a 'health-enabling community' is still in its infancy. HIV-related social researchers need to place far more emphasis on answering the following four questions: What constitutes a health-enabling community context? To what extent is it possible to create community contexts that enable sexual health? What are the factors likely to promote or hinder such an enterprise? How far can community-level interventions succeed in the absence of broader economic and political democratization in affected countries?

Against this background, there is a particularly urgent need to unpack the notion of community mobilization, and the associated concepts of grassroots participation and representation, and of multi-stakeholder partnerships. These concepts form the cornerstone of HIV-prevention programmes the world over, and are repeatedly cited as key strategies for building healthy communities. They have been echoed and re-echoed in a range of internationally subscribed declarations spear-headed by the World Health Organization.[20] Participation and representation are also the foundations of democracy, so this is a research question that has relevance way beyond the health and development arenas.

While the focus of this particular book is community mobilization for HIV-prevention, the mobilization of local people is necessary not only as a strategy for limiting the destruction of lives and families by limiting HIV-transmission, but also as part and parcel of how communities negotiate their response to the epidemic. In an attempt to deal with the impact, health care services increasingly have to ration the services they can give to people with HIV/AIDS.[21] Increasingly the burden of AIDS care is falling on households and communities. One frequently hears of lay people (nearly always women) nursing extremely needy and some-times difficult dying relatives with no medical support at all. Home-based care may take place in makeshift homes without running water, possibly without bedding, in a situation where dying patients may suffer from excessive vomiting or diarrhoea up to 15 times a day.[22] In addition to supporting those who provide such care, local community mobilization will also have to play a role in the distribution of drugs, once they become available to the more remote and hard-to-reach sectors. Thus, local community mobilization is not only a strategy for the *prevention* of further spread of HIV, it is also a key piece of the complex puzzle of how survivors of decimated communities can live through the epidemic, and come out of the other end of it as part of better, stronger societies.

## Introducing Summertown

The participatory community project in Summertown – the focus of this book – has sought to limit HIV-transmission through three activities: STI control (given that other STIs increase one's vulnerability to HIV-infection); community-led peer education and condom distribution; and local multi-stakeholder collaborative project management. The Project was initiated in the mid-1990s by a grassroots group of black African residents of a township in the gold mining region of Summertown, who came together because of growing local concern about HIV/AIDS. This group included local teachers, social workers, youth leaders, traditional healers and mine officials. A local government official introduced them to a group of academics (including the author of this book) who had independently approached an overseas funding agency for funding for an AIDS project. A lengthy process of negotiation brought together interest groups, which came to be called the Project's 'stakeholders'. These included the local grassroots group mentioned above, mine management, the trade unions, provincial and national government, and several researchers and international funding agencies. The stakeholders set up a non-governmental organization (NGO) to run the Project, employing three local Summertown-based full-time workers to accomplish this. It also employed a Johannesburg-based epidemiologist to co-ordinate the stakeholder committee, to mediate between the funders and the community, and to serve as Principal Investigator of the Project's large research component. The Project has been running since mid-1997, and the research in this book covers the period between mid-1997 and mid-2000.

Given the controversies surrounding the definition of the term 'community', it must be emphasized that, for the purposes of this Project, the term 'community' was defined as everyone living or working in the geographical area of Summertown. Summertown consists of a small formal town centre (formerly a white apartheid town) and a black residential township about 10 kilometres away. A little way out of the formal town are a series of gold mining shafts and twelve mine hostels in which migrant mineworkers live while performing their work contracts. Summertown is home to 170 000 predominantly black African people. About 70 000 of these are migrant workers on the gold mines, and most of the others live in the township. Gold is a key pillar of the South African economy, and mining jobs are highly valued despite difficult living and working conditions. Many rural areas in and around South Africa are totally dependent on mineworker remittances, and mining is the country's major source of foreign exchange. Migrant workers travel to the mines from a range of areas in and around South Africa, where they are housed in single-sex hostels, leaving their wives and families in their rural areas of origin.[23] The hostels, which sometimes house as many as 12 or 18 men in a room, offer no privacy and scant opportunities for intimate relationships. Within this all-male context, a thriving commercial sex industry has sprung up. Impoverished women find accommodation in informal shack settlements on mine perimeters from where they sell sex and alcohol to the miners who form the major consumers in a complex informal economy. Some women also sell sex in the veld surrounding the mine fences.

Most of the remainder of Summertown's residents live in a township in a range of housing types. About 65 per cent of residents live in small formal houses and 35 per cent in informal shacks made of corrugated iron and wooden poles. The township has benefited from some changes under the post-apartheid government, particularly an increase in the availability of formal housing. Other changes have been slower in coming. Township residents live with high rates of crime and violence (it is estimated that a woman is raped every 20 seconds in the province in which the township is located). Jobs are hard to come by as the local mines have suffered serious cutbacks over the past decade, and some of the jobs that do exist are less secure in a climate of increasing casualization of labour and the 'contracting out' of various tasks to outside companies.[24] Levels of unemployment are in the region of 40 per cent. Those who are employed often have unskilled and poorly paid jobs, and levels of poverty are high. A survey conducted in Summertown in 1999 found that among those who were employed the median income ranged from R1300 (GB£130) per month for miners, R1 000 (£100) for township men in other jobs, R300 (£30) for township women to R345 (£35) for women in the squatter settlements.[25]

Schools are underfunded, often battling with large class sizes, underqualified teachers and disappointing rates of school completion. South Africa continues to be a country characterized by dramatic social inequalities. A very small minority of young township people manage to find well-paid jobs in Johannesburg, but the vast majority do not. Many young people feel trapped in a community where they see few opportunities for their future advancement, and feel hopeless about their work prospects.

## The big picture: HIV/AIDS in South Africa

What is the broader context of HIV-prevention in South Africa? The epidemic reached the country a decade or so after Central and East Africa, providing a window of opportunity within which to implement appropriate prevention and management programmes. However, the apartheid government largely ignored HIV/AIDS and the post-apartheid government has not risen to the challenge of the epidemic, so that South Africa has become one of the AIDS capitals of the continent. Current estimates are that one in five adults, or a total of about five million South Africans, are living with HIV or AIDS, and 1 700 more are being infected every day.

The less affluent countries with the best records of success in limiting HIV-transmission include Thailand, Brazil, Senegal and Uganda. Each of these countries has dealt with the epidemic in its own way, but what they have in common is strong government leadership that has united various sectors of society in the fight against AIDS. The South African government, on the other hand, has become embroiled in a series of AIDS controversies resulting in disunity and conflict. For example, President Thabo Mbeki has done much to draw attention to the links between HIV and poverty in Africa, and between HIV and the legacy of apartheid in South Africa, a link that is well supported in the research presented in this book. However, he sought support for these views from widely discredited 'dissident' scientists who argue that HIV does not cause AIDS and even that AIDS does not exist as a specific clinical condition. The President's involvement in these debates has sown confusion among ordinary people trying to comprehend the nature and the extent of the epidemic, and has demoralized local health campaigners struggling to persuade a reluctant and sceptical public to practise safe sex. His involvement has created discord in local HIV/AIDS circles and despondency among local medical practitioners, health workers and academics. It has also drawn strong criticism from the church and the trade unions.

The country's National AIDS Plan, formulated in 1994 after much debate, represented a consensus among a range of interest groups from government, industry and civil society. However, the plan has never been implemented, partly because its authors were unrealistically optimistic about the economic and human resources that would be available for its implementation, and partly because government leaders failed to drive this process forward. While many South Africans are doing important work with regard to HIV/AIDS, the failure to implement the plan has marginalized many potential local AIDS experts and leaders, and their role has been taken over by international development agencies and externally funded NGOs. The country is awash with eager, jostling, overseas experts, often bearing large amounts of foreign funding. Too often, the language of HIV-prevention has become the language of western science and western policy approaches, not mediated by an appreciation of the extent to which these are inappropriate for local conditions. Externally funded project proposals may be written by overseas consultants and then handed over to local groups who have little sense of 'ownership' of the ideas in the proposals and who lack the organizational or technical skills, or the trained staff, to implement them properly.

Much research remains to be done on the dynamics underpinning the formulation of local HIV-related policies and interventions by non-local experts. One pioneering study traces the progress of policies for the treatment of STIs in South Africa.[26] These policies have been formulated by foreign academics and consultants, drawing heavily on scientifically rigorous research studies carried out in Tanzania and Uganda under the direction of experts mainly from developed countries. The study traces the process whereby such policies are communicated from international to national actors, and from the national level to the provincial clinics charged with implementing STI services. It highlights the myriad factors that have hampered implementation including, for example, the lack of 'fit' between policy recommendations and the reality of local conditions, where provincial clinics are under-resourced, lacking money as well as adequately qualified and motivated local staff.

In the following chapters attention will be drawn to a similar lack of 'fit' between the Summertown Project's well-intentioned and technically well-informed HIV-prevention proposal and the reality of local conditions in Summertown. In particular, while the proposal was an excellent one on paper, it was over-optimistic about the extent to which appropriate health systems and conceptual frameworks existed for pulling together the very diverse energies and talents of its stakeholders. The proposal was also optimistic about the ability and commitment of local stakeholders, doctors, scientists and industrialists, as well as grassroots community members, to implement a programme of such complexity.

## Synopsis of chapters

In addition to its introductory and concluding chapters, this book has four parts. Part I (Chapters 1 to 3) tells the story of the history and goals of the Summertown Project, as well as the background to the research presented in this book. Part of the impetus of the Project came from the author's baseline research into factors shaping HIV-transmission among gold mineworkers. This baseline research is the topic of Chapter 1, which highlights some of the factors shaping the sexuality of male migrant workers on the mines. It does so in the interests of highlighting why programmes that conceptualize HIV-prevention as an individual rather than a social problem are unlikely to have optimal impact, and why HIV-prevention activists are increasingly arguing for the types of community-level participatory approaches that informed the Summertown Project's design. Chapter 2 outlines the goals of the Summertown Project, with particular emphasis on the Project's commitment to implementing two methods of participatory HIV-prevention approaches that aim to create health-enabling community contexts – community-led peer education and stakeholder partnerships. The chapter concludes by outlining the nature of the evaluation research – on which this book is based – which seeks to evaluate the effectiveness of each of these participatory methods of HIV-prevention in the light of a study of the factors shaping sexual health in Summertown. Chapter 3 outlines the theoretical framework that guided the Project evaluation research, laying down the foundations of a social psychology of participation. (This is the most academic chapter of the book, and non-academic readers may wish to leave out this chapter, and go to the next one.) This framework conceptualizes the psycho-social and community-level processes whereby participation has its allegedly beneficial effects on health. Particular attention is paid to the concept of a 'health-enabling community', a community context that enables or supports the types of behaviour change that might reduce HIV-transmission.

Parts II and III provide detailed case studies of the social context of HIV-transmission and prevention – with particular reference to community-led peer education – among two of the Summertown Project's key participant groups: commercial sex workers (Part II) and youth (Part III) respectively. Each case study begins with a chapter examining the social construction of sexuality in its particular group of interest, with reference to the likelihood of condom use by members of the group. This is followed by an account of the Project's attempts to promote participatory peer education in each group, with a particular focus on the extent to which Project participants were able to implement effective peer education strategies within each context. Particular attention is given to examining the ability of peer education to promote the development of 'health-enabling community contexts' that support and enable the processes of individual and social change necessary for safer sexual behaviour.

Attention is also given to the extent to which local community-level strategies – such as peer education – have the potential to address problems that are often caused by macro-social problems whose roots lie beyond the borders of local communities. The two themes that recur repeatedly in both case studies relate to the way in which poverty and gender relations facilitate HIV-transmission, and undermine the effectiveness of HIV-prevention efforts. These chapters highlight the complex and challenging question of the extent to which the impacts of macro-social problems can be ameliorated by local community efforts.

To refer more specifically to each case study, the sex worker case study (Part II) is presented in Chapters 4, 5 and 6. Chapter 4 highlights the social construction of sexuality among Summertown sex workers. Almost seven out of ten women are HIV-positive. Detailed attention is given to the nature and context of the sale of sex, highlighting the way in which the construction of sex worker identities, within the context of women's particular working and living conditions, undermines the likelihood of condom use, and presents particularly severe challenges to participatory HIV-prevention efforts. Chapter 5 examines how women sought to rise to these challenges, creating a strong and united peer education programme in extremely unpromising conditions. However, the nature of their successes and failures, as well as the way in which a series of broader contextual factors undermined their efforts, raise numerous questions about the extent to which community-level programmes are able to redress problems that are fuelled by non-local social inequalities. These questions form the topic of Chapter 6.

The youth case study (Part III) is presented in Chapters 7 and 8. Levels of HIV infection are also high in this group, rising from 2 per cent for boys and 13 per cent for girls aged 15 to 35 per cent for men and 68 per cent for women aged 25.[27] Chapter 7 examines the way in which gender identities, constructed in conditions of severe poverty and lack of opportunity, often make the use of condoms particularly unlikely. Gender will have already emerged as a key determinant of sexuality in the sex worker case study (and indeed in the mineworker case study in Chapter 1). However, as will become clear, the mechanisms whereby gender impacts on the social construction of sexuality varies in the different life circumstances and daily survival challenges facing sex workers, mineworkers and youth, and for this reason it emerges as a key theme in each case study. Following discussion in Chapter 7 of factors militating against condom use by young people, in Chapter 8 attention is turned to the possibilities and limitations of school-based participatory peer education for addressing these challenges in the interests of creating contexts that enable and support the possibility of increased condom use. Attention is given to the possibilities and limitations of local community strategies (such as youth-led participatory peer education) to bring about behaviour change in the absence of long-term social development policies and interventions. Attention is also given to the institutional barriers to 'bottom-up' participatory projects. Ironically, Summertown Project workers found it far easier to mobilize the participation of grassroots people in the informal and chaotic contexts of sex worker squatter camps than it was in the relatively organized institutional settings of schools and gold mines.

In addition to peer education, the Project relied on a second participatory method of HIV-prevention. This was the method of multi-stakeholder partnerships, involving the collaboration of a range of local Summertown 'stakeholders' – including local government, the local mining industry, trade unions, grassroots groups, academic researchers and international funders – in project management. Part IV (Chapters 9 and 10) tells the story of this collaborative process, highlighting the complexities and challenges involved in pooling the very diverse talents and resources of so many disparate stakeholder groups. While the Project had some success in motivating stakeholders to work together in the fairly mainstream area of biomedical STI management, it had less success in mobilizing stakeholders to co-operate in the less familiar approach of peer education, and in collaborative project management by suitably representative stakeholders. Its greatest disappointment in the first three years of its life was probably its failure to promote widespread participation of mineworkers in project activities, either at the level of mineworker-led peer education or of adequate and appropriate mineworker representation on the project's stakeholder committee.

Two important factors are said to impact on the success of projects that rely on stakeholder partnership strategies. The first is the strength and quality of the partnerships formed by project stakeholder representatives. Part IV outlines various factors which undermined the quality of the alliance that the Project sought to forge between its stakeholders. These included a lack of understanding of the rationale for stakeholder collaboration, variable understandings of the causes of HIV-transmission and how to solve it, varying levels of stakeholder commitment to different project goals, and lack of trust among stakeholders. Dominated by biomedical experts, the stakeholder committee failed to develop adequate understandings of the social dimensions of the epidemic. It also failed to access appropriate expertise in the areas of health systems development, management skills and conflict mediation skills, which would have been necessary both to pull together the inputs of such a diverse array of stakeholders, and to deal with the personal and political conflicts that persistently undermined effective collaboration within the stakeholder group.

The second factor impacting on the success of community development projects is the extent to which potential grassroots project beneficiaries regard the project as relevant to their needs and interests. 'Grassroots project beneficiaries' include local township residents (including the majority of Summertown's young people), mineworkers and commercial sex workers, three groups living in situations that placed them at particularly high risk of HIV/AIDS. Part IV outlines how and why the representation of these groups on the stakeholder committee was non-existent at worst and patchy at best. Chapters 9 and 10 highlight ways in which the contact that did exist between grassroots people and other members of the stakeholder committee was often characterized by conflict and lack of trust. Part IV concludes by pointing to some of the practical lessons emerging from the Summertown Project's fraught attempts to pull together representatives of very different and often divided constituencies. Apart from practical lessons, it also seeks to make the more fundamental point that the deceptive neutrality of the term 'stakeholder' may serve to mask very real differences in the power that different stakeholding actors and agencies have to participate in, and to influence the course of, projects such as this one effectively. Part IV highlights how failure to take account of such power differentials severely impeded the potential effectiveness of the Project's attempts to form the collaborative 'partnerships' which feature so prominently in the rhetoric of politicians and development agencies whenever they outline appropriate strategies for fighting HIV/AIDS.

The concluding chapter of this book faces up to its findings. These are that the best-intentioned programmes, even when they achieve high levels of mobilization of the least-powerful sectors of small local communities, may have less than optimal results. This is because such programmes cannot succeed in the absence of the concerted efforts and commitment of more powerful members of society – locally, nationally and internationally – to develop innovative responses that are appropriate to the particular dynamics of the epidemic. The concluding chapter seeks to develop the notion of 'political will' to reveal how the best-intentioned project proposals may have a disappointing impact in the absence of both the commitment, the technical expertise and the organizational structures to implement complex and challenging programme proposals. As opposed to earlier studies, which refer to 'political will' as the will and commitment of formal government groups and politicians,[28] this chapter uses an expanded notion of 'political will', using the term to encompass a more complex range of micro- and macro-level sites in which power operates, including for example the most marginalized local communities, non-governmental organizations (NGOs), so-called local, national and international 'experts', multinational corporations and international development agencies.

International scientists and leaders are currently gaining much mileage from high-profile commitments to raising large sums of money for 'AIDS in Africa'. Much of this money is being earmarked for the development of biomedical responses, in particular drug treatments. Clearly, effective and accessible drug treatments have a vital role in reducing the immensity of the suffering of those already infected, and of their loved ones and carers. They also have a role in contributing to wider prevention efforts in various indirect ways. However, on their own, they neglect the needs of the majority who are not yet infected. In the absence of real commitment by national and international leaders to work towards creating community contexts that enable and support healthy behaviour, such money will be spent on Band-Aid solutions. Furthermore, while these solutions will serve the vital role of alleviating the suffering of many individuals and families in the short term, they will not change the community and social contexts that led to the development of the epidemic in the first place, nor will they strengthen affected communities in ways that will protect them from future hazards and future epidemics. The material presented in this book supports the argument that HIV/AIDS must be fought simultaneously on each of three time-scales: the short term (such as STI treatment, antiretroviral drugs), the medium term (such as community-led peer education and local partnerships to facilitate effective HIV-prevention and AIDS-care) and the long term (including measures such as macro-social policies and interventions that work towards the empowerment of women and poverty reduction).[29]

Given the enormity of these challenges in sub-Saharan Africa, where in areas such as Summertown HIV is a disease with a doubling time of just over a year,[30] advocating long-term macro-social changes alone offers cold comfort to those at most immediate risk of infection. Within such a context participatory community development approaches still have an important intermediate role, but there is an urgent need to understand and respond to factors that are most likely to promote and hinder their chances of success. Such approaches offer a better chance than individual-level interventions, but all those involved need to be realistic about the complexities of implementing these approaches, and the time they might take to produce measurable results.

The concluding chapter re-emphasizes the need for continued commitment to community-strengthening approaches to HIV-prevention as a vital complement to the energy and attention that are currently being given to the development and availability of treatments and vaccines. If treatments and vaccines are of vital importance, so too are vigorous prevention programmes that promote health-enabling community contexts. Despite the challenging complexities of implementing them, such programmes have the potential not only to change people's sexual behaviour but also to strengthen their collective ability to respond to health risks. The aim should be not only to achieve effective HIV/AIDS management, but also to build communities of survivors better equipped to face future unpredictable epidemics, and to reconstruct their life worlds once this particular epidemic has run its course.

# I

**The Summertown Project**
Context & Concepts

# 1

'Going Underground & Going After Women'

Sexuality & HIV-Transmission among Mineworkers

Research into the social construction of sexuality among migrant gold miners lent impetus to the development of the Summertown Project in the mid-1990s.[1] The aim of this research was to investigate why mining industry efforts to reduce sexually transmitted infections (STIs) and HIV-transmission through health education and STI clinics were having little impact. It was on the basis of these findings that the researchers argued that, on their own, mining industry programmes that conceptualized HIV-prevention as an individual problem were unlikely to have much impact, and that there was an urgent need to set up prevention programmes that also took account of the community and social dimensions of the problem.

The chapter starts with a brief history of the responses of both mine managements and trade unions to HIV infection up to the mid-1990s, as the context within which the interviews with mineworkers were conducted. This is followed by a discussion of the way in which miners' working and living conditions shaped their sexuality, and undermined their sexual health.

## Institutional responses to HIV/AIDS on the mines

The mining industry has been praised for the speed at which it implemented HIV-prevention interventions, long before either the apartheid or post-apartheid governments developed coherent responses to the problem.[2] This emphasis on disease prevention was a particular innovation for the mines, which traditionally had focused their efforts on tertiary rather than primary health care. However, mining approaches to HIV-prevention tended to rest on behavioural or biomedical responses. Behavioural responses took the form of information-based health education – which sought to persuade individual miners to change their behaviour, through providing them with factual information about health risks. Such approaches paid no attention to the way in which the social construction of sexuality would undermine the likelihood of such behaviour change by mineworkers, no matter how accurate their knowledge about sexual health risks. Biomedical responses took the form of the provision of STI clinics to treat diseases such as gonorrhoea and syphilis, which increase vulnerability to HIV. While these clinics were run by well-trained medical experts, they made no attempt to understand or accommodate the fact that miners' understandings of STIs, and the way in which miners sought treatment for STIs, were often not consistent with the biomedical model. In short, such approaches rested on individualistic western models of health and disease, aiming their efforts at individual mineworkers, with little attempt to understand or address the social or cultural factors that made mineworkers vulnerable to STIs and HIV.

Mine managements had persistently and explicitly denied any link between HIV/AIDS and social factors such as migrancy or single-sex housing, for example. This insistence that disease should be explained and treated at the level of the individual was clearly articulated by a South African Chamber of Mines' medical representative. She wrote of the 'profound gulf between those who come ... with an ideological perspective informed by a commitment to public health values and those whose views are informed by a primary commitment to the liberty of individuals as increasingly debated in the United States',[3] explicitly aligning the mining industry with the latter position.

Historically, mineworkers' trade unions had responded to HIV/AIDS through a focus on individual human rights – negotiating human rights policies and developing agreements with management around issues such as pre-employment testing and the prevention of discrimination against HIV-positive employees. While the unions had also made public statements seeking to link HIV/AIDS to factors such as migrancy and single-sex housing, these statements had not translated into significant pressure or action on the part of the unions. Unions had generally been reactive rather than proactive in relation to HIV/AIDS. In the few instances where unions had been involved in prevention activities, these had been initiated and funded by management or outside agencies such as non-governmental organizations (NGOs), and unions battled in the face of a lack of awareness of the urgency of HIV/AIDS among their members. Poor awareness of health risks among rank-and-file union members had long been cited as a problem facing trade unionists concerned with health and safety issues, even before the onset of the HIV epidemic.[4] HIV was proving to be no exception to this rule. While knowledge about HIV, its mode of transmission and its consequences had long been relatively high among mineworkers, the difficulty of organizing workers at the grassroots level around HIV/AIDS had been articulated by a number of union leaders.

There had also been a number of bipartite (management and unions) and tripartite (government, management and unions) meetings both nationally and internationally in the Southern African Development Community (SADC) region. These had resulted in a range of resolutions, policy declarations and codes, many of which were adopted unanimously by government, union and management delegates, often in agreement with similar tripartite groups from the surrounding countries with mining industries – such as Botswana, Namibia, Zimbabwe and Zambia.

However, there was no evidence that the biomedical, behavioural or individualistic responses preferred by the mining industry and the trade unions had made any impact on the epidemic among mineworkers. Clearly, human rights issues are vitally important, and the struggle to achieve these rights forms a key dimension of creating a climate that is supportive of people living with HIV/AIDS. Equally clearly, STI control and health education are important. Yet there was an urgent need to locate these efforts within frameworks that took account of the wider political, social, economic and development issues impacting on HIV-prevention, and to use these expanded frameworks to inform innovative prevention efforts.

## Miners' perceptions of health and HIV

At the time of the first set of interviews with mineworkers in 1995, levels of HIV among mineworkers were estimated to be in the region of 22 per cent, with heterosexual sex being the dominant mode of transmission. At the mine where the interviews were conducted, management was making strenuous efforts to educate workers about AIDS, with educational videotapes, pamphlets and posters. Preventive behaviour was also promoted through free supplies of condoms. Among the men interviewed, it was clear that these information-based programmes were having only a limited effect. Each man reported having seen the mine's educational videotape on HIV/AIDS; each was also aware of the pamphlets and posters providing information about HIV/AIDS and how to prevent it, and of the free supply of condoms. Every person said that HIV/AIDS was transmitted during unprotected sex, and that condoms would prevent its transmission. Most people said it was incurable. Beyond these basic facts, however, understandings of HIV/AIDS were patchy and often contradictory.

This study sought to illustrate the claim that knowledge about HIV/AIDS was more complex than a series of 'facts' of the kind that information-based health education programmes sought to impart (e.g. 'HIV is an incurable disease', 'condoms serve as an important means of HIV prevention'). The study sought to illustrate how these factors were located within a complex and detailed web of ideas concerning health, sexuality, traditional values and healing systems – with all of these ideas constructed in social conditions that shaped and constrained individual sexual choices.

Thus, for example, while miners were often in possession of the basic facts about HIV, which they had internalized through health education programmes, these facts were embedded within a range of doubts, qualifications, contradictions and uncertainties, which served to blunt the factual messages imparted by the programmes. Health education messages are not simply passively accepted by their audiences, but must compete with alternative beliefs, experiences and logics that may be more compelling than the information that the health educator seeks to impart. Many said that, while they had heard of HIV/AIDS, through the mine educational programmes and on the radio, they remained unsure about its existence because they had never seen anyone suffering from it.[5] Some people asserted that the disease did not exist, that it existed in countries to the north but not in South Africa, or that traditional healers could cure it. They cited the major symptoms of HIV/AIDS as sores on the body, and when asked to estimate the time lapse between infected sexual contact and appearance of sores, people often answered in the region of two weeks to two months. Most significantly, for all their exposure to the educational materials, unprotected sex with multiple sexual partners (frequently commercial sex workers) appeared not to be uncommon.

People articulated a notion of health that was more holistic than that of the biomedical model dominating western thinking about HIV/AIDS. They characterized health in terms of a harmonious balance between person and environment. The person was conceived of as an interaction of physical, mental and spiritual/supernatural imperatives. The environment included the living environment, working environment and social environment. They were comfortably located within a plurality of healing systems, moving between these without tension or sense of contradiction, oscillating between representatives of western biomedicine (hospitals, clinics, pharmacies, private general practitioners) and traditional healers (diviners, herbalists and faith healers).

Miners took the biomedically biased information they were given about HIV/AIDS (by people they saw as representatives of the western biomedical establishment), and interpreted it through a filter of health knowledge and experience in which western biomedicine played only a partial role. This filter led some to treat the claim that HIV/AIDS was incurable with a certain degree of scepticism:

> Interviewer: Is there anything that the traditional healers or western doctors can do to help, once one gets AIDS?
> Informant: Black people (traditional healers) can heal AIDS. AIDS is centred around sores, and black people are really good when it comes to healing sores.
> Interviewer: Can they eliminate it altogether?
> Informant: It is possible that they can eliminate the disease altogether if it is detected in its earlier stages.

A number of people claimed that one of the causes of 'the drop' (a colloquial term for gonorrhoea, one of a number of other STIs common on the mines and which increases miners' vulnerability to HIV) was sleeping with women who were taking the contraceptive pill. Another cause was sex with a woman who had recently taken some sort of traditional medicine in the interests of purging or cleansing the blood. The purgatives or the pill would leave 'dirt' inside the woman – which would then get into the male during sexual intercourse.

Informant: The drop is not a disease as such. It has to do with using the pill. It is the result of the dirt that comes from a person who is using the pill. If this dirt stays in you for a long time it develops into a disease.

Informant: You get the drop by sleeping with a woman who has drunk a potassium permanganate mixture to cleanse herself. All the dirt gets transferred from her into yourself.

For many people, traditional healers were considered the most skilled in dealing with this dirt. Mineworkers consult a wide range of healers without any tension or sense of contradiction. These include practitioners of western biomedicine, including hospitals, clinics, pharmacies and general practitioners in private practice, and traditional healers, including *sangomas* (diviners), *inyangas* (herbalists) and *umProfiti* (faith healers). Most people said they made use of both doctors and traditional healers for the treatment of STIs. They said they would first go to a biomedical doctor, who would give them an injection that took away the pain and 'put the disease to sleep'. However, biomedical treatment did not kill the 'eggs' that were the root cause of the problem. After this, they would visit a traditional healer who would administer an enema and other herbs that would, as one informant said, 'go inside of the person and take out the disease' and also generally purge the patient in the process.

Informant: The doctor's role is that he will give you instant relief with his injection. Thereafter the *inyanga*'s procedure must take place over a longer period. Firstly, you have to vomit after taking the emetic, then the healer will administer an enema, then you will take a steaming session to produce excessive sweat, and finally the healer will make incisions in your pubic area. All this process is some kind of cleansing of your reproductive system, and this gets rid of the 'eggs' that have caused the problem.

Some people said that one could go to a traditional healer and get preventive medicines, which would then 'block' these diseases (particularly STIs) from entering the person. Such treatment would make the use of condoms unnecessary.

Interviewer: How do you prevent getting an STI?
Informant: Before you sleep with a woman, you must drink manganese. This 'makgonatsohle' will kill any dirt from the woman that might have caused a disease.

Some mineworkers believed that supernatural factors played a role in the development of ill-health, with illness resulting from an enemy bewitching the victim, particularly by an acquaintance or relative who might be jealous of some good fortune the victim had experienced. In contexts where poverty and unemployment were high, jealousy of mineworkers' relatively well-paid jobs was not uncommon. One man explained his persistent bouts of gonorrhoea as the result of being bewitched by a neighbour in his home village. This neighbour, a former co-worker on the mines, was jealous that the miner had managed to retain his job during a bout of retrenchments, and that the miner's daughter had passed her school-leaving examination, which the former co-worker's daughter had failed. In such contexts, traditional healers play a key role in diagnosing and restoring the social disharmony that had led to the development of the disease.[6] Many mineworkers believed that, as soon as they learned that they were HIV-positive, they would simply have to consult those traditional healers who claimed to have a cure for AIDS. The traditional healers would then treat them with *muti* that would 'cleanse' the blood and flush the virus out of the system.

Having provided examples of some of the competing beliefs and ambiguities through which HIV education material was filtered by mineworkers, this chapter centres on two issues. The first concerns the particular set of working and living conditions that made unprotected sex with multiple partners such a compelling behavioural option for this group of migrants. The second concerns the interpretative frameworks used by people in accounting for their experiences of health, healing, sexuality and HIV/AIDS: it was these frameworks that formed the filter through which workers interpreted and responded to health educators' attempts to change their behaviours. It will be argued that miner identities, and their associated behavioural possibilities and constraints, are constructed in a way that makes them particularly vulnerable to HIV infection.

## Working and living conditions on the mines

Factors such as the general working and living conditions on the mines, the ever-present danger of accidents, and many men's perceived lack of control over their health and well-being are important features of the world in which mineworker identities are fashioned. Living and working conditions on the mines are dangerous and highly stressful.[7] Most mineworkers live some distance from their homes and families, in large single-sex hostels. Compound life is dirty and overcrowded, with no space for privacy or quiet – up to 18 people share a room. While some facilities exist for visiting wives and families, people said that these were extremely limited. Opportunities for leisure are few. Some workers spend time in the African townships near to the mines; others avoid them as dangerous places. Drinking and sex are two of the few diversionary activities easily available on a day-to-day basis.

Even more stressful than life outside of work, however, is the time spent in the mines themselves. While miners' working conditions vary widely according to their specific job underground and according to the demands of particular production team leaders (who, some people commented, sometimes seem to be more concerned with productivity than with the well-being of the team), there are many common themes. Many men said that they were expected to engage in physically taxing and dangerous work for up to eight hours with infrequent breaks, sometimes with minimal access to food or water. They spoke of working conditions of tremendous heat, in air that was frequently stale and dusty, and sometimes with unpleasantly noisy machinery in narrow sloping tunnels.

In talking about the stresses of daily life on the mines, the threat of rock falls emerged as the central concern of most of the people interviewed. They spoke of living in daily fear of fatal, mutilating or disabling accidents. This fear was well founded. The South African mining industry has long been characterized by an alarming accident rate.[8]

> Informant: Every time you go underground you have to wear a lamp on your head. Once you take on that lamp you know that you are wearing death. Where you are going you are not sure whether you will come back to the surface alive or dead. It is only with luck if you come to the surface still alive because everyday somebody gets injured or dies.

> Interviewer: Do you worry about death from accidents, working underground?
> Informant: This thought scares us when something has happened – maybe to a person one knows, or even a person one does not know. You might hear that so-and-so has gone (in an accident) and you think: 'Eish! our brothers are passing away', that's all. We cannot know, maybe we are also on the way, and we live in hope – and with the knowledge that it will happen to everyone sooner or later. We live for dying, no one lives forever. Every day people lose their arms and legs and we just live in hope.

Many had witnessed accidents in which friends and co-workers had been either killed or injured, or had seen the dead or injured being brought above ground after accidents, and the stress and distress caused by such incidents cannot be underestimated. The psychologically disabling effects of being subject to life-threatening or shocking incidents are well documented in the literature on post-traumatic stress, as is the fact that, while some are able to make a quick recovery, others suffer the after-effects for varying periods after the incident. This study's interviewees included members of the latter group. They reported the classic symptoms of post-traumatic stress disorder following the trauma: social withdrawal; problems concentrating; and flashbacks or nightmares in which they relived the shocking incident. Such flashbacks or nightmares sometimes troubled them for months or even years after the accident. Several people talked about the disturbances at night caused by the screaming of men suffering nightmares, who would then be woken up and comforted by room-mates.

Men referred to accidents in a fatalistic way.

> Informant: The rock can just fall anytime and we try not to think about that. A rock can fall and kill someone while you are working with them, it has

happened to me before ... last week someone in my team met his fate that way and we had to pull his corpse from under the stones.

Interviewer: Are there any religious measures that people take before starting to work?

Informant: No one prays or does such things – because when a rock is going to fall it just falls anytime and there is nothing that can be done about it.

Interviewer: Is there any form of traditional protection that people seek out – to try to protect themselves against falling rocks?

Informant: There are those that seek help from traditional healers for protection, but when the rocks fall, they fall all over, and it does not matter whether you are protected or not – they fall on those with and without the protection.

This sense of powerlessness is an important feature of the contextual backdrop against which miners' sexual identities are negotiated. Self-efficacy (or the degree to which a person feels that he or she has control over important aspects of his or her life) is an important determinant of health-related behaviour. The greater one's sense of self-efficacy, the more likely one is to engage in health-promoting behaviours.[9] It was not only in relation to accidents that people referred to a sense of powerlessness. In the interviews, they repeatedly articulated their lack of control in a range of contexts. For example, virtually every interviewee said he hated his job, but that he had no choice given his lack of education, and the high levels of unemployment and chronic poverty in his rural place of origin.

Interviewer: Is your job easy or difficult?

Informant: The work is heavy but I have endured it because I have no education. It's risky – every time I go down I am not sure if I will come back. But I have no choice. I am forced to do it.

Interviewer: Would you say that this is a source of pride for these men that they do this dangerous and difficult job?

Informant: Facing such struggles is not a source of pride. It is because of frustration and poverty that men do this job.

Many commented on their powerlessness to avoid a range of health problems. Tuberculosis (TB) was one such problem.[10] One 25-year-old man said it was inevitable that if he stayed on the mines for twenty years he would get TB, no matter how much he tried to avoid it. A 41-year-old man who looked considerably older than his years appeared depressed and apathetic. Speaking about his recurrent bouts of TB, he said he was pessimistic that he would ever be in good health again.

Interviewer: Given the situation you working in, are there any attempts that you make to improve your health?

Informant: There is nothing that I try because I don't have that privilege. Where I am living on the mines, I don't have any choice on how to conduct my life, it is imposed on me. Most of my life that I have spent here has not been so fruitful, and when I look ahead, I don't see myself having a long life.

Interviewer: Why do you say that?
Informant: Because of my ill-health and I don't spend a year without visiting a hospital.
Interviewer: Do you not feel that this negative attitude might encourage you to be lazy about looking after yourself?
Informant: I care about my life very deeply, but I can really feel that I am suffering with my health – I feel that my life won't last for much longer, and that due to my working conditions I am prevented from prolonging it.

While people spoke with feeling about frightening working conditions and poor living conditions, they had little faith in their ability to bring about improvements. Complaints to unions or *indunas* seldom bore fruit. One man commented wryly in response to a question about channels for complaint:

Interviewer: Is there any way you can complain about things you do not like?
Informant: There are several channels for complaints, but we are never considered. So, we just complain for the sake of complaining.

One informant commented that the risk of HIV/AIDS appeared minimal compared with the risks of death underground, and suggested that this was the reason why many mineworkers did not bother with condoms.

Interviewer: Why is it that men think about pleasure first before thinking about their health?
Informant: The dangers and risks of the job we are doing are such that no one can afford to be motivated with life – so the only thing that motivates us is pleasure.

Having pointed to features of the social context within which mineworkers construct their identities, attention is now given to the interpretative frameworks drawn on by mineworkers in presenting their health-related life histories. Such repertoires shape not only sexual behaviours, but also responses to HIV-education programmes that attempt to change sexual behaviours.

## Health, intimacy and sexuality

Masculinity emerged as a central theme structuring mineworkers' accounts of their health-related experiences and behaviours.[11] Attention is given to the way in which the social construction of masculine identities on the mines makes migrant mineworkers especially vulnerable to HIV infection. Much has been written about the creative and innovative way in which mineworkers have responded to the alienation and danger of their working lives, constructing personally meaningful identities despite massive social constraints.[12]

Particularly evident in the interviews was the way in which masculine identities had been shaped and crafted by workers as a way of dealing with the fears and struggles of their day-to-day working lives. Men frequently spoke of their terror as new workers the first time they entered the 'cage' (lift) that would carry them to their work sites as much as three kilometres underground. They recounted how more experienced workers would encourage them by urging them to remember that they were men. A man was someone who had the responsibility of supporting his family, and hence had no choice but to put up with the risks and stresses of working underground. A man was someone who was brave enough to withstand the rigours of the job.

> Interviewer: How did they console you when you entered the cage?
> Informant: They told me that in this situation you must know that now that you are on the mines you are a man and must be able to face anything without fear.
> Interviewer: Is this theme of being a man common in the mine?
> Informant: To be called a man serves to encourage and console you time and again…. You will hear people saying, 'a man is a sheep, he does not cry'. I mean, this is the way to encourage or console you at most times.
> Interviewer: Can you explain more about the metaphor of 'a man being a sheep'?
> Informant: I can explain it this way: no matter how hard you hit a sheep or slaughter it you will not hear it cry. The animal that can cry is a goat. So, that is a comparison that whatever pain you can inflict on a man you will not see him cry.

Thus the notion of masculinity plays a key role as a coping mechanism whereby men overcome their daily fears of injury and death as well as the exhausting demands of the work. As one informant told me: 'We commit ourselves as men because if we don't do it our children will suffer.' Another commented:

> You show your manhood by going underground, working in difficult conditions – this shows that you are man enough to accept that if you die you are just dead. Once you go underground you are a man and no longer a child.

Closely intertwined with this notion of masculinity – which brings together the concepts of bravery, fearlessness and persistence in the face of the demands of underground work – is that of a macho sexuality, which was captured in another informant's comment: 'There are two things to being a man: going underground, and going after women.' Linked to this masculine identity were the repertoires of insatiable sexuality, the need for multiple sexual partners and a manly desire for the pleasure of what is locally called flesh-to-flesh sexual contact. All these are factors that put mineworkers at risk of HIV/AIDS. Ironically, the very sense of masculinity that assists men in their day-to-day coping also serves to heighten their exposure to the risks of HIV infection.

Interviewer: Why do you think that men have sex on their minds?

Informant: I think that is the way men were made, that is to always have a desire for a woman.

Interviewer: You have a family that you love and support, but on the other hand you behave in a way that can make you vulnerable to diseases. Why should men behave like that?

Informant: The truth is that 'a man is a dog', meaning that he does not get satisfied. That is why we come across such things. Because when a man sees 'a dress', meaning a woman, he follows her.

Interviewer: Why do people think about pleasure before they think about their life which is at risk?

Informant: The truth is that we are pushed by desire to have sex with a certain woman. We do not think about AIDS during that time but about it when we are finished. It is a matter of satisfying your body because of someone beautiful. Basically it is the body that has that desire.

People made a strong link between sex and masculinity in relation to their general physical and mental health and well-being. Particularly important for health was what was referred to as the maintenance of a balanced supply of blood in the body. Several people commented that sex played a key role in the regulation of a balanced supply of blood and sperm, and that regular sex was essential for the maintenance of a man's good health. They mentioned a range of possible ill-effects of poorly regulated bodily fluids resulting from prolonged celibacy. People dwelt most on mental ill-effects: depression, short-temperedness, violence and an inability to think clearly. Less frequently mentioned were physical ill-effects including pimples and obesity. Behavioural ill-effects included recklessness and impulsive behaviour. A normally prudent and responsible man who had been celibate for too long might, it was claimed, be unable to control his desire for sex when he encountered a commercial sex worker in the street, even if he did not have a condom with him. Lengthy celibacy might also lead a man to consider homosexual relationships that he would not have considered in other circumstances.[13] Unrequited sexual urges might also lead a man to take unnecessary risks in the African townships near the mines, by seeking out women whose friends or brothers might beat him up or steal his money.

The continued practice of dangerous sexual behaviours by mineworkers must also be located within a context that provides limited social support and scant opportunities for intimacy. Research in both Europe and America has found a significant correlation between level of social support and safe sex. People are less likely to engage in unprotected sexual intercourse if they live in a supportive social environment. In conditions where they felt lonely and isolated, flesh-to-flesh sexual contact may often come to symbolize a form of emotional intimacy that is lacking in other areas of their lives.[14] Safe sexual behaviour is predicted more by teenagers' perceptions of how much their parents care for them than by the frequency of health warnings, social class or parents' health status.[15]

This correlation between social support and risk-taking behaviour provides an interesting framework within which to consider the high levels of unsafe sexual behaviour practised among mineworkers. Men spoke at length about the loneliness of being away from their families. They spoke of anxieties that their distant rural wives or girlfriends might be unfaithful, of worries about their children growing up without a father's guidance, of their own guilt about money they might have wasted on drink and commercial sex, which they should have sent to their families. These absent families were never far away in their accounts of their lives and their health. Others spoke with dread of fears that they would die underground, and that their bodies might not be returned to their families for proper funeral rites, a particularly frightening prospect in a context where deceased ancestors may often play a pivotal role in people's lives.

While hostel room-mates, underground team-mates and men from the same home village appeared to constitute support systems in certain contexts, miners were adamant that male friends could not make up for the loss of female partners and children within a homely domestic setting. The youngest informant (aged 19), and also the most sexually active and least interested in condoms, spoke wistfully of his close relationship with his parents in rural Lesotho, and how much he missed them. The 41-year-old interviewee referred to earlier, who had been plagued by recurrent attacks of tuberculosis for five years, gave his distance from his wife as one of the main reasons for his poor health.

> Informant: There is no one who can help me here, and it is quite impossible for me to know all my needs. If I were nearer to my wife, she would take care of me, look after me.

In response to questions about their reluctance to use condoms, miners repeatedly reiterated their desire for flesh-to-flesh contact. When asked specifically about the reasons for this desire, people referred to pleasure, and also to the fact that this was simply something that men needed: 'a man must have flesh to flesh' was something of a cliché in the interviews. Research findings cited above suggest that another reason for the desire for flesh-to-flesh contact might be the broader social context of general loneliness and reduced opportunities for intimate social relationships.

In the highly patriarchal rural communities from which many mineworkers come, one of the main pillars of masculine identity is participation in homestead and family leadership.[16] In the particular context of life on the mines, deprived of such key markers of masculinity on a day-to-day basis, frequent assertion of what are regarded as healthy and manly sexual urges could arguably serve to compensate for reduced opportunities for assertion of masculine identities in other contexts.[17]

The material obtained from these interviews illustrates the complexity of automatically viewing high-risk health-threatening behaviours in a negative light. It has been suggested that risk-taking is better conceptualized as a 'wager', in which social actors weigh up potential losses and gains of the behavioural options available to them.[18] While mineworkers may be aware of the dangers of unprotected sex with multiple partners, such behaviour may be beneficial at a range of other levels in the stressful and socially impoverished living and working environments of the mines.

## Reframing the debate: Towards a discourse of 'enabling approaches'

The interview findings echoed the call for a shift in the discourses that shape sexual health promotion campaigns, away from biomedical and behavioural interventions and towards so-called 'structural interventions'[19] and 'enabling approaches'.[20] Rather than trying to *persuade* people to change their behaviour through education programmes, or through encouraging them to attend STI clinics, such approaches turn their attention to the possibility of creating circumstances that *enable* behaviour change. They focus on the social and environmental determinants that facilitate or impede behavioural choice, and aim to remove structural barriers to health-protective action as well as constructing barriers to risk-taking. Tawil and colleagues illustrate their argument with a review of the context of HIV-transmission in developing countries, arguing that enabling approaches should focus on the economic development of at-risk groups, as well as on development policy. Through a focus on the powerlessness of many women to protect themselves against HIV-infection, they look at a range of economic and policy strategies aimed at improving women's access to resources, and their subsequent financial dependence on male partners who are unwilling to use condoms for a complex mix of reasons.

In the interests of justifying the need for the Summertown Project, these interview findings were used to argue that the existing 'top-down' approaches of mine management urgently needed to be supplemented with participatory approaches that sought to promote the 'bottom-up' involvement of mineworkers in designing and implementing programmes. Furthermore, biomedical and behavioural models – which conceptualized HIV-prevention at the level of individual change – needed to be supplemented with community development and policy approaches that conceptualized HIV-prevention at the level of community and social change. Such an approach would mean that prevention efforts should target not only mineworkers, but also members of the broader communities in which miners conducted their social and sexual lives. It would also require the gold mines to work hand in hand with local health departments, as well as seeking to collaborate with a new and less conventional series of partners including local grassroots community groups, traditional healers and sex worker representatives. Inspired by the discourse of creating 'enabling community contexts', the Summertown Project sought to conceptualize HIV/AIDS in a way that moved beyond individualistic perspectives.

## 2

**Mobilizing
a Local Community
to Prevent HIV/AIDS**

The Summertown Project

The Summertown Project was a large community-led HIV-prevention intervention in a mining community near Johannesburg. It was initiated by a partnership between a local township grouping concerned about levels of HIV/AIDS in Summertown and some academics,[1] who had independently approached an overseas development agency for funding for an AIDS project on the basis of the research outlined in Chapter 1. A lengthy process of negotiation resulted in the formation of the Project stakeholder management team (including the local group, mine management, trade unions, provincial and national government, donor representatives and several researchers), who set up a non-governmental organization (NGO) to run the Project and employ three full-time workers.

The Project rested on the assumption that three sets of activities were most likely to bring about a reduction in HIV. The first was the aggressive syndromic management of sexually transmitted infections (STIs) – this was the state-of-the-art STI control measure at the time the Project was established. The second was community-led peer education and condom distribution. The third was the establishment of a multi-stakeholder committee, representing a partnership uniting key community constituencies, which would oversee Project management. This approach to project management was a change from traditional mine programmes. The Project would be managed not only by mine managements, as was usually the case, but by an alliance of management, trade unions, grassroots community organizations, academics and funders, and representatives of the provincial and national health services.

For reasons discussed in the next chapter, the active involvement of this very diverse range of stakeholders would be essential if the Project were to have any hope of success in addressing the way in which Summertown people's working and living conditions placed their sexual health at risk. All the stakeholders participated actively in meetings leading up to the establishment of the Project, supported the establishment of the Project and pledged their commitment to it. One of the themes of this book is the varying extent to which stakeholders followed through this early nominal commitment in the form of concrete action towards achieving Project goals. Attention will be given to the way in which the apparently neutral 'stakeholder' concept (a well-established concept in the development lexicon) masks very real differences in the power of diverse groupings to influence the process of collective projects, and in their motivation to engage in genuinely collaborative action with other groups.

The involvement of stakeholder representatives in the Project's management was one of a series of strategies that sought to improve on existing interventions in ways that took account of the context of sexual activity more broadly than traditional HIV-management programmes had in the past. The Project was to be aimed not just at mineworkers but also at members of the surrounding communities, in which miners conducted their social and sexual lives. Attempts would be made to involve a wide range of traditional and biomedical practitioners in Project activities, in line with many Summertown residents' commitment to both health systems. Rather than relying on information-based HIV-education, community-based outreach and peer education strategies would be used. Every effort would be made to ensure that target audiences participated as fully as possible in the design and implementation of these strategies. Such participation would provide the context for a critical renegotiation of sexual norms, and for increasing workers' sense of self-efficacy in relation to their health, both of which were seen as essential preconditions for behaviour change.

Community-based peer education programmes were designed with the explicit goal of moving beyond the limitations of information-based education programmes. Clearly, knowledge of health risks is a key precondition for health-enhancing behaviour change. However, as argued earlier, imparting knowledge about how to avoid health risks needs to go hand in hand with creating contexts where people are most likely to put that knowledge into action. The Project was designed in a way that sought to view HIV-transmission as a community problem rather than simply as an individual problem. This would involve seeking not only to improve the health-related knowledge, motivation and behavioural skills of individual mineworkers, but also to create community contexts that would be supportive of mineworkers transforming such knowledge and skills into health-enhancing behaviour. It also sought to maximize networking between this local initiative and other HIV-prevention initiatives at a provincial and national level, in the interests of strengthening local efforts.

From the outset, there was an awareness of the difficulties of implementing a project of this nature. In an article written in 1998, project researchers emphasized the challenges facing the Project.[2] One shortcoming would be that it could not extend its activities to the rural areas in the range of southern African countries where many migrant workers have their homes. Thus while miners' town communities, and their town girlfriends and partners, would be exposed to the intervention, their rural girlfriends and partners would not. The success of the Project would depend on the density of networking among all the Project's different stakeholders at community, provincial and national levels. The extent to which this networking was possible remained to be seen. Furthermore, Project outcomes would depend on whether national efforts to develop multi-sectoral HIV-prevention policies got off the ground in South Africa. Local industry-based initiatives would have the best chance of success if they were located within supportive national and provincial policies, which would, it was hoped, serve to reinforce the impact of work done at the local level.

Speaking more generally, a project of this nature asks the controversial question: can health be improved without eliminating the wider social inequalities that provide the contexts in which ill-health so often flourishes? Those with the poorest health experiences the world over are generally those who come from the most disrupted social settings, and are the least constrained or protected by family and community expectations; HIV in South Africa is no exception to this general rule. Ideally, the most important aspect of slowing down the spread of STIs and HIV infection in Summertown would be to alter the broader social and material conditions that encourage high-risk sexual practices.[3] These would include measures such as an end to the rural poverty that makes it necessary for people to migrate to work and the provision of full employment for all. They would also include an end to the gender inequalities that often mean that women are both psychologically and economically ill-equipped to insist on condom use in the face of reluctant men, or to resist abusive relationships that place their sexual health at risk. However, such changes involve ongoing long-term struggles. Given the lack of widely affordable and accessible HIV drugs and vaccines, and the speed at which the epidemic is progressing in South Africa, additional short-term strategies (such as STI control) and medium-term strategies (such as community-led peer education) are required to deal with HIV. The challenge for HIV educators remains urgent.

Community participation, a central pillar of the Project and the focus of this book, is a key medium-term strategy. Empirically, there is evidence that community-led approaches (including peer education and multi-stakeholder management) have had some successes in marginalized populations in some countries and contexts – even in the absence of broader macro-social changes.[4] Furthermore, within marginalized communities, there are individual differences in ability to take control of health, with some people or families being better equipped than others to respond to health campaigns.[5] Politically, many people (including many African feminists) have argued against the tendency to view poor people or women as passive victims of paralysing macro-social forces beyond their control, incapable of acting to improve their lives. Conceptually, there is a sound case to be made that social changes of the kind needed to address the HIV epidemic are best achieved through a combination of top-down and bottom-up struggles. Such an understanding of social change underpins the argument that, in principle, community-led health-promotional networks provide the potential for ordinary people to add their voices and contribute their views to debates about the kinds of social changes that need to be made, and how best to implement these.

The Project's overseas funding agency commissioned a London-based consultancy company to develop the Project proposal. This company contracted a highly respected, but non-local, specialist in HIV-prevention to write a proposal based on his experiences in a range of other African countries. In retrospect, having an outsider write the proposal was less than ideal for a number of reasons. The first was that it meant that local stakeholders had a limited sense of ownership of the original ideas of the Project. Although there was some consultation between the external consultant and some Summertown stakeholders in the development of the proposal, this appears to have been fairly superficial. During the course of implementing the Project, key Project actors and stakeholders were not always familiar with the proposal or with the Project goals or rationale outlined in it. Use of outside experts to formulate Project plans also has the potential to reinforce a passive attitude among local people, and to generate a sense of disempowerment and even apathy, playing in a culture of believing that challenging problems are best solved by 'overseas experts'. Furthermore, the 'log frame' procedure that the proposal provided to guide the process of project implementation (outlining project aims, inputs and outputs) was complex and difficult to understand. As a result it played a minimal role in helping local people to implement the proposal.

## Who are 'the Summertown community'?

A key unresolved issue that bedevils the academic literature on community development is what constitutes a community, and what is the best way of demarcating the most appropriate unit of focus for community projects. Some speak of communities of place. Others speak of communities of interest or communities of identity, which are not necessarily geographically bounded. These might include particular religious or special interest groups such as the gay or anti-globalization communities, whose members do not necessarily live or work in one geographical space, or necessarily know one another.

Operating under severe logistical, resource and organizational constraints, HIV-prevention programmes in poor countries have tended to focus their energies on geographically defined communities. As outlined in the introduction, the 'Summertown community' referred to in the Project proposal consisted of a geographical region including the small formal Summertown city centre, the large adjacent township that housed the majority of Summertown's residents, the gold mines and their hostels scattered around the formal town, and the small informal squatter camps from which sex workers operated. Associated with this geographical community were a variety of groups with very different identities, interests and motivations, as well as very different degrees of access to economic and political power and resources.

From the outset, within the Summertown Project discourse, the term 'community' was used in a confusing way to demarcate two groups with very little overlap. On the one hand, in relation to Project management and leadership, the Summertown community included representatives of the formal constituencies that had an economic or professional interest in health or wealth in the geographical region of Summertown. These included the gold mines, the mineworker trade unions, the provincial and national health departments, an overseas development agency and a group of academics. It was representatives of these groups who constituted the Project's 'stakeholder committee'. While all these groups did indeed have an interest (or 'stake') in Summertown's economic or general well-being, in practice many stakeholder representatives were based in the head offices of these constituencies rather than in their local Summertown offices. Particularly in the first two years of the Project's life, most of the stakeholder committee members were based in the cities of Johannesburg and Pretoria, about an hour's drive from Summertown, rather than being drawn from the local Summertown branches of these constituencies. Members of this group were generally considerably more affluent and educated than the average Summertown resident. Furthermore, more than half of them at any one time tended to be white, compared with the actual residents of Summertown, who were overwhelmingly black. It was this rather élite stakeholder group that was implicitly regarded as the *managers* or *agents* of change.

The term 'community' was also used interchangeably in other contexts to refer to the relatively poor, and less influential, mass of grassroots Summertown residents (particularly miners, sex workers and young people). This group was implicitly regarded as the *target* of change, and for various reasons was not represented or under-represented on the stakeholder committee.

The Project's effectiveness was severely undermined by this schizophrenia about who constituted 'the community' that would have to undergo change if the Project was to succeed in limiting HIV-transmission. The stakeholder committee operated on the implicit assumption that its role was to exercise leadership in the task of getting the so-called 'target groups' (particularly miners, sex workers and youth) to change their behaviour and practices. There was never any sense among the leadership group that their own behaviours and practices might also have to change in order to address the problem. This failure by powerful stakeholder groups to acknowledge that they too were part of the community, and would need to change along with everyone else, seriously undermined the potential effectiveness of the Project's achievements.

## What is peer education?

Three groups of strategies or approaches are most commonly used within health promotion: information provision, self-empowerment and collective action.[6] Information-provision approaches seek to increase people's knowledge about the causes of health risks and how to avoid them. Information is transmitted through such channels as school lessons, counselling by health professionals, the mass media, leaflets or posters. Such approaches are didactic in nature, involving the transmission of information from an outside expert to a passive target audience. They are based on the assumption that people engage in unhealthy behaviour owing to ignorance. Once they are in possession of correct information they will allegedly change their behaviour, since individuals are conceptualized as rational decision-makers whose cognitions inform their actions.

A second group of health promoters has argued that, in addition to providing people with *information*, it is necessary to increase individuals' *motivation* to perform healthy behaviours, as well as training them in the appropriate *behavioural skills*. The so-called self-empowerment approaches seek to address all three dimensions, with the aim of empowering individuals to make rational health choices through strategies to increase their motivation and behavioural control over their physical, social and internal environments. Such approaches are based on the assumption that every individual has the power to act in ways that protect his or her health, and that the role of health promoters is to help people identify that power and teach them how to use it. Self-empowerment approaches might work with young people to motivate them to resist peer pressure to smoke or to have unwanted sex, by developing their psychological resources to 'say no' – through methods such as assertiveness training or social skills training. In relation to sexual health, such approaches may involve rehearsal with target groups of communication scripts or interactive sequences involved in condom purchase or sexual negotiation with a condom-averse partner.

As already stated, however, the best information-provision or self-empowerment approaches are unlikely to change the behaviour of more than one in four people – generally the more affluent and educated members of a social group. This is because health-related behaviours are not always under the conscious rational control of appropriately skilled and motivated individuals. They are also determined by the extent to which community and societal contexts enable and support the performance of such behaviours. In unequal societies, where material, social and psychological resources are unequally distributed, individuals do not always have the power to put healthy choices into practice.

This presents health workers with the challenge of developing policies and interventions that aim not only to provide people with information, motivation and behavioural skills at the individual level, but also to promote the development of social and community contexts that enable and support the performance of health-enhancing behaviours, through the so-called collective action approaches. Within the context of the collective action genre, the concepts of grassroots participation and community mobilization have emerged as key conceptual tools in the *practice* of health promotion. Community-led peer education, a central pillar of the Summertown Project, falls within the 'family' of collective action approaches.

Peer education is one of the most commonly used strategies of health promotion throughout the world, particularly with young people and hard-to-reach groups.[7] In the HIV arena, peer education involves training members of groups who live and work in situations that place them at high risk of HIV-infection to disseminate information about sexual health risks, and to distribute condoms. Ideally, community members play a key role in the selection of their peer educators. This is to ensure that peer educators are seen to be representative of the groups that they serve, and have the respect that will assist them in playing their leadership roles. Peer educators are given basic knowledge about sexual health, as well as training in participatory health educational skills, such as dramas and role-plays. Peer education is based on the assumption that people are most likely to change their behaviour through collective action to change peer norms. As such, it offers an improvement on the self-empowerment approaches, insofar as it shifts the locus of behaviour change from the individual to the peer group, acknowledging that sexuality is shaped and constrained by collectively negotiated peer identities, rather than simply by individual-level information, motivation and behavioural skills.

While peer education programmes have had some success in some countries and contexts, this is not always the case. Shifting the level of analysis from the individual to the peer group level is often not enough. The peer groups that are often the most vulnerable to poor sexual health (such as sex workers or young people) are also those that have the least power to challenge the environmental factors undermining their sexual health. As a result, some peer education programmes are located within the context of a broader community development approach, with much emphasis placed on strategies such as 'women's empowerment' or 'community strengthening'.[8]

Such approaches may include equipping prospective peer education participants, drawn from groups who may not have had the experience of working co-operatively within organized settings to meet mutually beneficial goals, in team-building and organizational skills. They may also include the development of leadership skills among groups of women, who might never have had the opportunities to exercise leadership in strongly male-dominated communities. Such programmes often also seek to promote women's economic empowerment programmes and to reduce women's economic dependence on men who might refuse to use condoms. They may also seek to link up peer groups from marginalized communities with more powerful groups at the local and national level, in an attempt to mobilize support for project goals.

The Summertown Project used the peer education approach developed by the Project Support Group (PSG) at the University of Zimbabwe. The PSG's model of peer education has been used successfully in a number of southern African countries.[9] As a regionally appropriate method that had earned both national and international support and respect, the PSG model was chosen as the 'gold standard' for the Project. The support that the PSG offers peer education projects has three stages. First, prospective peer education co-ordinators visit the PSG head office in Harare, Zimbabwe, for training. Thereafter, they are sent back to their regions with written support materials that consist of ten 'training module' booklets. Each of these provides a detailed outline of the various stages involved in setting up, conducting and monitoring a peer education project. Novice peer educator co-ordinators use these modules to guide them through the process of setting up new peer education programmes in their areas. Lastly, the PSG continues to offer support and guidance in the wake of the training process. PSG experts periodically visit the new peer educators on their home turf, observing the activities they are implementing, and offering support and advice. The PSG also organizes regular meetings to bring together their peer educator trainees from various regions, providing them with a context in which they can offer one another support and advice.

Presented in an easily accessible form, the ten PSG modules are designed to guide grassroots groups through all the stages of setting up, conducting, monitoring and evaluating a peer education programme. Early modules focus on how to set project goals and how to conduct formative research within the local community, focusing on issues such as identification of local groups at highest risk of HIV infection, the physical locations where members of these groups can best be reached by peer educators, the extent of group members' capacity for participation in peer education programmes, the specific nature of their educational needs and so on. Such information forms an essential input into strategic planning by peer educator leaders. The modules also include detailed guidance on how to implement participatory approaches for HIV-prevention. These include strategies such as role-plays, dramas and easy-to-implement picture cards for promoting debate and discussion of issues relevant to sexual health. Modules also include what are referred to as 'quality assurance' guidelines – in the form of checklists that help peer educators to ensure they are providing factually accurate messages, and outlining procedures for the organization and conduct of project meetings. Guidelines are also provided for the field support of peer educators, for the monitoring and evaluation of peer education programmes, and for the financial management of programmes. Over a number of years, PSG workers have put a huge amount of care and thought into presenting modules in a way that is easily accessible and logical to people who might not have high levels of literacy or organizational experience.

## Project evaluation research: Outcomes and processes

In the overall Project management strategy, two forms of evaluation were used. First was *outcome* evaluation, which sought to measure changes in HIV and other STIs before the start of the intervention, and then at various stages during the life of the intervention.[10] Second was *process* evaluation, which sought to explain the processes underlying programme successes or failures.[11]

The Project's outcome evaluation research was conducted by a group of epidemiologists and biomedical researchers, and took the form of an ongoing series of quantitative surveys measuring a range of biomedical, behavioural and social factors on a random sample of 2 000 people every year. There were ongoing delays in the analysis of the Project's impact data, and key HIV-prevalence data are still not available. However, the partial outcome evaluation of the Summertown Project conducted to date shows that, within the three-year period of interest, the Project had no measurable impact on levels of chlamydial infection, syphilis or gonorrhoea, or on the proportion of people who had experienced a genital sore in the past 12 months.[12] If the Project had been successful in increasing condom use and improving the uptake of effective STI services, one would have hoped for reductions rather than increases in STI levels. This lack of impact was evidenced in the three groups surveyed (sex workers, mineworkers and township residents aged between 15 and 49). Indeed, among mineworkers, far from being a reduction in STI prevalence, there was actually a significant increase in the prevalence of all three of these STIs, and in the proportion of mineworkers with a genital sore in the past 12 months.

The Project's process evaluation research, co-ordinated by the author of this book, ran from 1995 to 2000. This took the form of ongoing in-depth interviews with Summertown residents, Project workers and stakeholders; and an analysis of Project documentation, including Project policy documents, minutes of monthly stakeholder meetings and a number of consultancy reports that were commissioned by the Project's various funding agencies over this period to record and assess various aspects of Project functioning. It is hoped that the Summertown experience may yield useful insights for future programme planners in the area of community-led HIV-prevention, as well as generating debate about possible measures that future projects might take to increase their likelihood of success.

Although some of its activities (STI control, health education and condom distribution) were fairly typical of HIV-prevention programmes on the mines, the Summertown Project departed radically from traditional mining industry programmes through its emphasis on two forms of local community participation. The first was its promotion of community-led peer education among mineworkers, sex workers and young people – the three groups in Summertown whose living conditions made them particularly vulnerable to HIV infection. The second way in which the Project departed from traditional mining industry initiatives was through its aim of facilitating the involvement of, and partnership among, the wide range of local community representatives (the 'stakeholder' committee) in collaborative project implementation.

In this chapter, the goal of maximizing local community participation is put into context within broader debates about health inequalities. Then a framework for conceptualizing the processes by which participation has the potential to impact on the health of community members is outlined.[1] A large international literature points to the way in which a combination of two forms of social disadvantage – material social exclusion (poverty) and symbolic social exclusion (lack of respect and recognition) – are key determinants of poor health in many countries and contexts in both the North and the South. The pathways along which social disadvantage impacts on health are many and complex. Apart from the direct effects of socio-economic deprivation on health, members of marginalized groups often lack the material or symbolic resources to deal with health-damaging stress. Social exclusion often undermines access to health-related knowledge. Furthermore, people who lack the power to shape their life course in significant ways – through poverty and/or through low social status – are less likely to believe that they can take control of their health, and thus less likely to engage in health-promoting behaviours.

Those who seek to reduce the impact of social disadvantage on health pit their energies at various levels. Some work at the level of governments, some at the level of NGOs. Others seek to promote partnerships between the public and the private sector, and still others work to formulate and implement health-promoting social policies at the global, national, regional or local levels. Some work directly in the areas of health. In the current climate of 'joined-up thinking', others work to create alliances between health activists and representatives of social sectors that impact on health in more indirect ways, such as welfare, housing, transport, women's issues, education and employment.

Each of these levels of struggle forms an essential backdrop for the interest in community development and participation – which are regarded as one component in a toolkit of strategies for improving the health of disadvantaged groups and communities. Within the area of health promotion, in particular, recent years have seen 'a paradigm drift' away from biomedical and behaviourally oriented interventions and policies towards a community development perspective.[2] This perspective is driven by the insight that the impact of health programmes is likely to be maximized by the participation and representation of grass-roots communities in planning and implementation.

Various arguments are made for the importance of participation in health, either directly or indirectly. First, there is growing recognition of the need to involve local community groups in strategic and operational decisions about health service design and delivery. This is deemed crucial for addressing issues such as differential access, cultural differences, racism and communication difficulties, which are often believed to undermine the level of health service provision received by marginalized groups in various countries and contexts. Second, it is argued that local community groups should participate in the design and implementation of campaigns to promote health-enhancing behaviour change – through methods such as community-led peer education, since people are far more likely to change their behaviour if they see that liked and trusted peers are changing theirs. Third, there is an argument that recognizes the more indirect but equally important influence of local community/ neighbourhood conditions on health, with studies emphasizing that social cohesion and strong local networks benefit health in a number of indirect ways. For this reason health promoters are increasingly seeking to involve themselves in general 'community-strengthening' programmes that seek to create 'health-enabling communities' characterized by trust, mutual support and high levels of involvement in local community projects of mutual interest. Multi-stakeholder partnerships, between a wide range of diverse community groupings in the interests of meeting collaborative goals, are regarded as a key means of strengthening communities and creating a health-enhancing environments.

Yet, despite the growing emphasis on participation among those concerned with health inequalities, much remains to be learned about the pathways by which participation and representation have a positive impact on health and community development. Despite the key role participation plays in the *practice* of public health, in both health policy prescriptions and health intervention designs, *theoretical* development in this area is weak. As a result, the ability to learn lessons from successful and unsuccessful participatory programmes is limited. Taking peer education as an example, this approach is now the method of choice for sexual health promoters working with 'hard-to-reach' groups in both rich and poor countries.[3] Yet while some peer education programmes have been successful in promoting health, others have had disappointing outcomes. Understanding of the processes and mechanisms underlying their successes or failures is still in its infancy. Recently, peer education has been described as 'a method in search of a theory'.[4] It has been argued that peer education 'suffers from an inadequately specified theoretical base, which does not address the important social and cultural factors implicit in the approach',[5] and that this gap undermines the possibility of learning from its successes and failures.[6] The participatory method of multi-stakeholder partnerships suffers from a similar lack of theoretical underpinnings.

One reason for this shortcoming relates to the difficulty in theorizing practical interventions. There is often a lack of communication between health and community development workers in real-life social settings, on the one hand, and researchers and theoreticians in universities, on the other. One of the key goals of the Summertown research was to bridge the theory–practice divide through an in-depth longitudinal study of attempts to promote community participation for health using the two participatory strategies of peer education and multi-stakeholder partnerships for project management. This chapter points to some of the conceptual tools for a 'social psychology of participation', which seeks to highlight the psycho-social and community-level mechanisms by which participatory approaches have their allegedly beneficial effects on health. It is this framework that informed the investigation of the Project's community mobilization efforts. In particular attention is given to the four interlinked concepts of social identity, empowerment and critical consciousness, social capital and power.

## Social identities

Social identities consist of those aspects of one's self-definition that arise from membership of particular social groups (e.g. occupational groups such as mineworkers or sex workers) or from one's position within networks of power relationships shaped by factors such as gender, ethnicity or socioeconomic position. Different identities or positionings are associated with different behavioural possibilities or constraints (recipes for living). Rather than being static, permanent or given, social identities are constantly constructed and reconstructed from one moment to the next. This process of construction takes place within social contexts that enable or constrain the degree of agency that people have to construct identities or to behave in ways that meet their needs or represent their interests.

In contrast to traditional views that health-related behaviours are determined by individual rational choice, the social identity literature emphasizes how health-related behaviours are shaped and constrained by collectively negotiated social identities.[7] Thus, for example, using a condom or visiting a traditional healer is an act structured by social identities rather than simply by individual decisions.

The past decade has seen a drift away from formal didactic health educational methods towards participatory approaches within HIV-prevention. This change in practice has gone hand in hand with a conceptual shift away from understanding 'sexual behaviour' as the product of individual decisions, in favour of the concept of 'sexuality' as a socially negotiated phenomenon, strongly influenced by group-based social identities and more particularly peer identities. Peer norms are seen as the result of a process of collective negotiation by young people in peer group settings. Ideally, the peer education setting should be a microcosm of 'the thinking society',[8] a term that refers to the way in which social identities and their associated recipes for living are collectively shaped through a combination of debate and argument in everyday-life contexts.

Traditional didactic health education seeks to change the views and attitudes of isolated individuals. By contrast, peer education seeks to bring about changes at the level of the peer group. In peer discussions, individuals' inputs weave and clash through the process of dialogue and argument between peers, as they ask one another questions, exchange anecdotes and comment on one another's experiences and points of view. Ideally, peer educational settings provide a forum where peers can weigh up the pros and cons of a range of behavioural possibilities, developing accounts of alternative behavioural norms and options in their own terminology and in light of their own priorities.

Social identities play a key role in the processes whereby unequal power relationships (such as relationships between men and women) are reproduced or transformed. Identities are constructed and reconstructed within a range of structural and symbolic constraints that often place limits on the extent to which people are able to construct images of themselves that adequately reflect their potentialities and interests. So, for example, female identities are often constructed in ways that predispose women to collude with men in sexual relationships that do not necessarily meet their needs and interests.[9] These may include practices such as forced sex, or sexual relationships that prioritize male pleasure over female pleasure and well-being. Ideally, peer educational settings should provide a context within which a group of people may come together to construct identities that challenge the ways in which traditional gender relationships place their sexual health at risk. In such a situation, social identities become potent tools for social change. Successful participation in collective community projects provides an important context for the reconstruction of social identities in health-enhancing ways.

The potential success of participation is influenced by the degrees of freedom that people have to construct new and empowered identities. In more affluent countries, identity theorists have emphasized the fluid and changeable nature of the process of identity construction in late modern (or post-modern) societies.[10] They place much emphasis on the importance of avoiding unduly essentialist accounts of identity. Essentialism is said to arise when one provides universalistic or over-generalized accounts of the content of identity categories such as 'masculinity' or 'women', for example. Such generalizations allegedly fail to take account of the variety of ways in which men and women are said to construct and transfer these identities from one situation and context to another. Situations of chronic material and symbolic marginalization sometimes limit the opportunities that people have to shape alternative identities (the existence of which is taken for granted by many theorists located in more affluent countries). There is still much to be learned about the possibilities and limitations of participation in contexts where poverty and gender inequalities limit the potential for the reconstruction of alternative social identities by deprived groups.

## Empowerment and critical consciousness

The renegotiation of collective identities within peer education settings needs to happen in conjunction with the development of peer groups' confidence and ability to act on collective decisions in favour of health-enhancing behaviour. Much work has been done on the role of empowerment in shaping health-enhancing behaviour change. Such work starts with the assumption that powerlessness or a 'lack of control over destiny' severely undermines the health of people in chronically marginalized or demanding situations. Disempowered people, who have little control over important aspects of their lives, are less likely to feel that they can take control of their health.[11]

Understanding of the concept of empowerment varies. Some writers have emphasized the role that psychological empowerment plays in promoting the performance of health-enhancing behaviours. This is a fairly superficial notion of empowerment, which implies that people can be empowered as individuals through methods such as assertiveness training courses. Others have been fiercely critical of the psychological reductionism inherent in this understanding of empowerment. Critics argue that psychological empowerment cannot take place without real political and economic empowerment. Unless participatory health promotion programmes are accompanied by real changes in the access that participants have to symbolic power (defined in terms of perceived respect and recognition from others) and economic power, they are unlikely to succeed.

Many debates about empowerment focus on the *emotional* or *motivational* dimensions of empowerment, conceptualizing it in terms of a subjective sense of confidence. Paulo Freire's conceptualization of empowerment adds a more *cognitive* or *intellectual* dimension to understandings of empowerment, focusing on people's intellectual analyses of their circumstances. Freire argues that a vital precondition for positive behaviour change by marginalized social groups is the development of 'critical consciousness'.[12] The Freirian notion of critical consciousness involves the two interlinked dimensions of understanding and action. The first aspect of critical consciousness involves development of group members' intellectual *understanding* of the manner in which social conditions have fostered their situations of disadvantage in ways that undermine their health. In terms of Summertown, this would involve some kind of intellectual understanding – by participants in HIV-prevention programmes – of the way in which factors such as poverty and gender shape the poor sexual health experienced by local people. It is this intellectual understanding that constitutes an important precondition for *action* – for groups to work together to challenge or resist some of the adverse social circumstances that place their health at risk.

Thus, for example, a successful peer education programme might provide a group of men with the opportunity to discuss the way in which the construction of masculine identities increased their risk of poor sexual health. They might further discuss the way in which the achievement of conventional masculine identities was limited by poverty and unemployment. In South Africa, unemployed men aiming to take on the male breadwinner role and set up their own families are constrained when they lack the money to buy houses or pay a *lobola* (bride-price). They may over-compensate by adopting an overly macho and controlling attitude to women in sexual relationships. From a Freirian perspective, such understanding would form the starting point from which men could collectively work towards redefining their masculinity in ways that were less endangering of their sexual health, and acting on this newly developed understanding.

According to Freire, the development of critical consciousness involves people moving through a series of stages. The first is 'intransitive thought', characterized by 'naïve' rather than 'critical' consciousness. At this stage people lack insight into the way in which their social conditions undermine their well-being, and do not see their own actions as capable of changing these conditions. Through a gradual process of deepening critical insight, the process of participation ideally leads to the final stage, that of 'critical transitivity'. This stage is characterized by the dynamic interaction between critical thought and critical action that may result when people learn to think critically about their life situations. Such a critically transitive thinker is empowered to reflect on the conditions that shape his or her life, and to work with similar others to change these conditions on the basis of such critical insight.

According to Freire, the transition from naïve to critical consciousness involves an 'active, dialogical educational programme'[13] in which participants are actively included in formulating critical analyses and generating scenarios of alternative ways of being. However, he warns that a range of obstacles stands in the way of people benefiting from such a programme. In particular, life situations characterized by exploitation and oppression lead to the development of 'adapted consciousness' rather than critical consciousness. Adapted consciousness refers to a state where 'a person accommodates to conditions imposed on them, and acquires an authoritarian and a-critical frame of mind'.[14] This constitutes a situation of 'democratic inexperience' within which disadvantaged people have a limited ability to conceive of alternatives to existing social relations, let alone the confidence to challenge such social relations.

Within a Freirian framework, an important goal of peer education is to provide a context for the development of people's critical consciousness about their sexual health. It should do so through stimulating the development of insight into the ways in which social relations, particularly gender relations constructed within conditions of poverty, undermine the likelihood of good sexual health. It should also stimulate the development of the belief that existing gender norms can be changed, as well as scenarios for alternative ways of being. It is on the basis of such critical thinking that a group of people is most likely to engage in collective action to challenge social relations that place their health at risk.

## Social capital

A 'health-enabling community' refers to a social and community context that enables or supports the renegotiation of social identities and the development of empowerment and critical consciousness, which are important preconditions for health-enhancing behaviour change. There is currently much controversy about how best to conceptualize such a community, with the concept of 'social capital' featuring in many debates in this area. According to the social capital approach, people are most likely to undergo health-enhancing behaviour change if they live in communities that offer high levels of participation in local networks and organizations, which are associated with increased levels of trust, reciprocal help and support, and a positive local community identity.[15] It has been argued that that the most important dimension of health-enhancing social capital is 'perceived citizen power'.[16] This is a characteristic of communities where people feel that their needs and views are respected and valued, and where they have channels to participate in making decisions in the context of the family, school and neighbourhood.

Recently, much attention has been given to the possibility that the concept of 'social capital' might provide an integrative framework for conceptualizing those features of community most likely to enable and support health-enhancing behaviours.[17] It has been argued that people are more likely to be healthy in communities characterized by high levels of social capital. Along these lines, it has been argued that an important determinant of the success of participatory health-promotional interventions is the extent to which they mobilize or create social capital. Social capital is considered to be important for health promotion for two reasons. First, communities that are rich in social capital are said to provide a supportive context within which people can collectively renegotiate social identities in ways that promote the increased likelihood of health-enhancing behaviours. Second, residents of communities with high levels of social capital are most likely to have high levels of perceived control over their everyday lives. This is important for health, given that people who feel in control of their lives are, in general, more likely to take control of their health, through either health-enhancing behaviours or the speedy and appropriate accessing of health services. These points resonate with insights from the work on empowerment and critical consciousness. Furthermore, most importantly, a critical conceptualization of social capital is one that takes account of the complex series of linkages between marginalized local communities and more powerful groups. The quality and quantity of these links play a key role in enabling or constraining the potential success of health-promotional interventions.

The notion of social capital has taken strong hold in the discourse of leading international development agencies, and the task of building or enhancing local social capital is increasingly regarded as a key dimension of a range of health-promoting development initiatives in disadvantaged settings. However, the concept has also roused fierce criticism for its failure to take account of the way in which various forms of social exclusion undermine the possibility of creating, sustaining or benefiting from social capital in marginalized communities.[18] Critical social scientists have expressed concern that a focus on community-level determinants of health could serve to displace attention from the well-established links of health, poverty and racism.[19] The controversy about the concept of social capital has mostly taken the form of a polarized argument about the relative benefits of community-level (i.e. social capital) and macro-social (e.g. racism, poverty) explanations of health.

It is argued here that neither community-level nor macro-social determinants of health can be understood without reference to the other. Community-level factors will often play a key role in mediating between social disadvantage and health. Thus, for example, poverty is clearly a primary cause of health inequalities, and the economic regeneration of deprived communities is essential for reducing such inequalities. However, if one of the effects of poverty is to undermine health-enhancing community networks and relationships, *economic regeneration* must be accompanied by *social regeneration* (i.e. projects to enhance social capital) if they are to have optimal success in improving health.[20]

Concern has been expressed that concepts such as social capital and participation are dangerously ambiguous.[21] On the one hand, they serve as potential tools for critical social theorists who argue that it is only through grassroots participation in strong community-based organizations that socially excluded people will gain the power to lobby governments and other powerful bodies to recognize and meet their needs. On the other hand, such concepts have the potential to be 'hijacked' by neo-liberal, free market theorists, who argue that grassroots organizations and networks have the power to take over many functions (e.g. welfare) previously assigned to governments or international development agencies.[22] Such arguments can serve as justifications for cuts in welfare spending in the more affluent countries of the North, and reduced development aid to poorer countries in the South. In order to avoid this perversion of the radical potential of the concept of social capital, it is vitally important that critical social scientists locate conceptualizations of social capital, participation and community development against the backdrop of wider conceptualizations of politics and power.

The concept of social capital has generated great enthusiasm, and is now used in a range of contexts, with a range of definitions. Within the public health arena, it has been argued that the concept has become so vague and imprecise that it is in danger of losing its analytical edge.[23] In the interests of guarding against such imprecision, in this book, the concept is used very specifically to refer to participation or 'civic engagement' in local community networks, with particular emphasis on local people's participation in the community-led HIV-prevention networks of the kind that the Summertown Project sought to create. Such participation is said to be associated with increased levels of trust, reciprocal help and support, and positive local identities.

A great deal of the writing and research in the social capital tradition tends to portray social capital as an overwhelmingly positive social resource, and one that is freely available to local communities irrespective of the extent of their social disadvantage. Yet evidence suggests that not all forms of local participation have equally positive benefits for participants.[24] Furthermore, there is much evidence that social capital is often unequally distributed in particular contexts. Thus, for example, research has shown that effective participation in local networks is most likely to take place among the wealthiest and the most educated members of a community.[25] Furthermore, social capital may often serve as a source of social exclusion and disadvantage, in contexts where opportunities for creating, sustaining and accessing beneficial social capital are constrained by poverty, or other forms of social inequality, such as caste or gender.[26]

## Towards a critical conceptualization of social capital: The double-edged nature of power

In contrast with the wide range of authors who have talked about social capital in an atheoretical and descriptive way, detached from any broader theory of society,[27] Bourdieu emphasizes the role played by different forms of capital in the reproduction of unequal power relations.[28] He argues that unequal social relations are maintained through a range of social processes that sustain inequalities in the interlocking phenomena of economic capital, human/cultural capital and social capital. It is Bourdieu's conceptualization of the role played by social capital in reproducing or transforming social inequalities that forms the basis of the research in this book. Social capital is conceptualized in terms of people's participation in mutually beneficial social networks that underpin collective action in the interests of pursuing mutually beneficial goals (in this case, the goal of reducing HIV-transmission). Particular attention is given to the way in which the Summertown Project's attempts to build social capital were enabled or hindered in the divided and unequal power relations that characterize South African society, of which Summertown is a microcosm.

The Summertown research into the participatory community development approaches of peer education and multi-stakeholder partnerships attempts to capture the dialectic of enablement (grassroots community agency: the empowerment of local people) and constraint (structural obstacles: resistance to change by powerful groups; unequal power relations between local stakeholders) that characterizes the process of participation. Often, at the very moment that local programmes open up the tantalising possibility of the empowerment of local people to take control of their sexual health, they simultaneously come up against a series of institutional barriers to such change. This is illustrated by the way in which Summertown Project's attempts to promote strong and successful grassroots initiatives involved the constant negotiation of the ever-thin line between the sphere of possibilities and the sphere of limitations. Again and again the Project highlighted the ambiguous way in which poor people are simultaneously *subjects of* their own lives, yet *subject to* forces beyond their control.

Drawing on the classic work of Hannah Arendt,[29] Jovchelovitch has pointed to the need for a 'double-edged' conceptualization of power to accommodate this complex dialectic of enablement and constraint.[30] On the one hand, she highlights the power differentials between groups who have unequal access to the material and symbolic resources most likely to assist them in collectively working for conditions that best enable them to pursue their needs and interests. The research in this book will show, for example, the way in which a combination of gender relationships and poverty made it difficult for female sex workers to assert their interests when interacting with male mineworkers, undermining the success of sex worker-led peer education efforts. It will also show how project attempts to increase young peoples' confidence and capacity for critical thought were hampered in a more general context of impoverished living conditions, poor educational and career prospects, divided families and communities, and a hierarchical and authoritarian school system. It also highlights the limited power of small NGOs (such as the Summertown Project) to influence the world views and practices of more powerful groups such as the trade unions or the mining industry (whose support would have been essential for the implementation of those aspects of the programme involving mine worker participation). Different social groups hold different levels of power to participate in constructing life projects that meet their needs and interests. Jovchelovitch argues that participation in conditions where material and symbolic obstacles prevent the possibility of real social change can be a hollow exercise. It legitimizes the status quo rather than providing an opportunity for marginalized people to pursue their needs and interests.

On the other hand, conceptualizations of power must also allow for the possibility of empowerment. 'Power is not a phenomenon to be explained only through an intrinsic negativity, but as a space of *possible action*, where social subjects strive to exert their effects.'[31] Power is inextricably linked to that realm where people collectively participate in the everyday negotiations bringing different social groups and identities into dialogue about the possibility of social change. 'Power, in this sense, is deeply intertwined with participation. It refers to being capable of: to be able to produce an effect, to construct a reality, to institute a meaning.'[32] Whenever a community participates in activities and initiatives to enhance its interests, it actualizes the power it holds to participate in the shaping of its way of life.

Social change through participation can be properly understood only if one understands the ambiguity of power relations and the double-edged nature of power. The dialectic of constraints and possibilities is the motor of social change. Social scientists have a role to play in unpacking the mechanisms implicit in this process if they hope to contribute to the development of actionable theorizations of the role of participation as a public health strategy.

## Participation, power and the (im)possibility of social change?

The four concepts of social identity, empowerment/critical consciousness, social capital and power consitute the starting point for the development of a 'social psychology of participation', which seeks to outline the processes underlying the successes or failures of participatory HIV-prevention strategies, such as peer education or multi-stakeholder project management.[33] This task is informed by a critical conceptualization of identity construction. Social identities are constructed and reconstructed within a range of material and symbolic constraints, which often place limits on the extent to which people are able to construct the images of themselves and their claimed group memberships that fully reflect their potentialities and interests. However, at particular historical moments, often through participation in collective projects and networks, members of socially excluded groups may indeed come together to construct identities that challenge their marginalized status. In some circumstances, participation may take the form of participation in networks of collective action, which serves either directly or indirectly to improve people's material life circumstances, or raise the levels of social recognition they receive from other groups. Within such a context, social identities and participation have the potential to serve as important mechanisms for social change.

However, there is evidence that participation in local networks is most likely to take place among the most advantaged members of a community, so it could be argued that measures to increase local community participation could have the unintended consequence of perpetuating social disadvantage rather than reducing it. For this reason, it is vitally important that policies and interventions advocating participation as a means of addressing social inequalities should not be blind to the complexities of seeking to promote such participation by socially excluded groups.

## 'Partnerships' in community development: Bonding and bridging

Within the context of a desire to move beyond individualistic biomedical and behavioural policies and interventions, the concept of social capital has been cited as an important tool for focusing attention on a range of community-level factors (such as grassroots participation), which are believed to play a key role in the success or failure of health-promotional efforts.[34] Kreuter argues that one important determinant of the success of health-promotional interventions lies in the extent to which target communities either have, or develop, organizational systems and networks that support the intervention, and the extent to which these are activated. The activation of these organizational entities depends partly on the extent to which people are aware of them, identify with them, value them and trust them. In this context Kreuter defines social capital as 'those specific processes among people and organizations, working collaboratively and in an atmosphere of trust, that lead to the accomplishment of goals of mutual social benefit'.[35]

Putnam[36] distinguishes between two forms of social capital, which provides a useful starting point for conceptualizing the nature of the local community relationships that might contribute to the development of a health-enabling community. The first is *bonding* social capital, which refers to exclusive, inward-looking social capital located within homogeneous groups. Such social capital bonds people in relationships characterized by trust, reciprocal help and support, and a positive common identity ('within-group' social capital). This is the kind of social capital that might arise from the development of close-knit, sex-worker, peer-education groups, or the strengthening of particular youth peer groups that have a commitment to HIV-prevention. Bonding social capital links individuals together within strong horizontal peer groups, resulting in the benefits and resources that accrue from close trusting relationships with similar others.

Putnam's second category is called *bridging* social capital, and refers to links that occur between social groups ('between-group' social capital). This is the kind of social capital that links diverse groups with varying levels of access to material and symbolic power. Bridging social capital brings people in contact with the resources and benefits that accrue from having a wide and varied range of social contacts. These social contacts exist as a valuable resource for the different groups involved. They are associated with trusting and supportive relationships among groups of people whose world views, interests and access to resources might be very different, but who have some sort of overlapping mutual interest (e.g. in HIV-prevention).[37]

The importance of bridging social capital in relation to HIV-prevention is based on three interlinked assumptions. The first is that epidemics arise when existing methods of managing diseases are inadequate. In other words, dealing with an epidemic involves the creative establishment of new approaches and new alliances that are specifically tailored to the new demands presented by the epidemic disease in question. The second assumption is that 'the whole is greater than the sum of the parts'. Not only is the HIV epidemic too complex to be dealt with through traditional biomedical or behavioural disease prevention. It is also too multi-faceted for any single constituency (e.g. provincial clinics or local grassroots people) to deal with on its own. For this reason it is essential that HIV-prevention projects build alliances with the widest possible range of relevant constituencies, to ensure that a wide range of actors pool their resources and creativity in working to create a new approach that is relevant to the precise manifestations of the disease in question. This takes us to the third assumption, that the relationships between different groups of actors do not take place on a level playing field.[38] Different groups have very different access to resources and influence. The concept of bridging social capital draws attention to the importance of ensuring that traditionally isolated and disadvantaged groups (such as sex workers) are put in touch with vertical networks of influence and expertise (including appropriate public and private sector networks and policy-makers), whose support may often be vital if they are to maximize their own efforts to promote their interests and well-being.

This bonding/bridging distinction is useful for clarifying those forms of participation and collaboration that are most likely to further the goals of community-led HIV-prevention projects in ways that take account of the double-edged nature of power. It is through the development of bonding social capital that a group of people takes the first step towards developing a critical consciousness of the material and symbolic obstacles to their health and well-being, and begins to develop both the insight and the confidence to address these obstacles. The promotion of strong bonding social capital within a group of marginalized people (e.g. sex workers or young people) is most likely to provide the starting point for the renegotiation of identities, as well as the processes of empowerment and critical consciousness, which are the essential first step for the success of participatory peer education, for example.

However, in addition to promoting bonding social capital through approaches such as peer education, for example, it is equally vital that community development projects promote partnerships between local peer education networks and other appropriate groupings (from civil society, government and the private sector) in the development of three forms of bridging social capital in order to elicit the support they may need to challenge these obstacles.

First, programmes need to maximize the development of bridges between small local community groups (sex worker or youth peer groups, for example) and more powerful local groups (such as the local mining industry or local teachers' associations) who have the local-level power and resources to assist them in their quest to develop more health-enabling community contexts.

The second form of bridging social capital links small local groups into networks of influence beyond their geographical location. These include the development of bridges (such as national sex worker or youth associations), which may serve as a medium through which small local peer groups are able to add their voices to extra-local debates about regional and national policies and interventions that support their local efforts. According to Paulo Freire, a key dimension of successful participation includes the development of opportunities for small local groups to become involved in social change projects that aim for change beyond their immediate community contexts. He argues that the activity of participation is most likely to be successful when it enables people to take part in collective action aimed at changing themselves, their local communities and the wider societies in which they live, simultaneously.

The third form of bridging social capital (sometimes referred to as 'linking social capital'[39]) involves links between small local groups and more powerful extra-community groups or agencies in the political, economic, medical and donor spheres, whose support might be vital to the success of their activities.

## 'Communities' and 'stakeholders'

One of the key goals of the 'social psychology of participation' is to open up space for a critical conceptualization of the nature of the 'community' that makes up the subject of 'community development' and 'community participation'. What are the boundaries of the 'communities' within which participatory programmes seek to promote the possibility of health-enhancing behaviour change – through the reconstruction of community members' social identities in more health-enhancing ways, the development of their critical consciousness of the obstacles to behaviour change, and the promotion of a sense of collective empowerment or agency to challenge these obstacles, and the facilitation of appropriate forms of bonding and bridging social capital?

For a range of logistical reasons, so-called community development projects in less affluent countries and settings most frequently define a community as the inhabitants of a particular geographically defined area.

Yet this definition of community has been widely criticized by those who point out that people who live in the same area do not necessarily constitute a community.[40] Rather than defining communities in terms of common area of residence, critics argue that a community is a social psychological construct, with the essential defining feature of a 'community' being a sense of common identity among a group of actors, or a sense of common interest in achieving particular goals.[41] The failure of many community development projects is often explained in terms of the failure of development agencies to acknowledge the frequently divided and conflictual nature of relationships between people living in particular geographical areas.[42] Such failure is also often ascribed to the naïve assumption of development agencies that it is possible to instil a sense of collective commitment to a common project among individuals or groups, simply because they occupy a common geographical space.

In the past few years, some development practitioners and agencies have attempted to acknowledge the complex and contested nature of local communities through the growing popularity of the concept of the 'multi-stakeholder community'. The recognition that geographical areas are often home to a range of different 'stakeholders' represents an important first step towards acknowledging the frequently diverse nature and interests of local groups and actors. This is only a first step, however. In the field of HIV-prevention, further conceptual development work still needs to be done in two respects. First, more work needs to be done to conceptualize the different types of relationships within and between local stakeholder groups, with a view towards deepening understanding of the way in which these relationships serve to support or hinder the goals of participatory HIV-prevention programmes. Second, more emphasis needs to be placed on the fact that relationships between diverse local stakeholder groups seldom take place on equal terms. Unequal power relations between different groups may impact heavily on their ability to influence the process of stakeholder collaboration, and their motivation to participate in genuine collaboration with other stakeholder partners.

While the Summertown Project focused its efforts on those who lived and/or worked in a geographically defined space, it sought to take account of the complex array of relationships within this space through its acknow-ledgement of the importance of both bonding and bridging relationships and its emphasis on peer education and multi-stakeholder collaboration. It was through peer education that the Project hoped to promote strong collective action within homogeneous peer groups of particularly vulnerable groups such as sex workers or young people (bonding social capital), in the interests of reducing HIV-transmission. Further, there was recognition that the efforts of marginalized groups would need to go hand in hand with the collaborative efforts of a number of diverse and more powerful stakeholder groups (including private sector, public sector and civil society groups) in order to achieve these goals (bridging social capital).

A key theme in the case studies that follow is the way in which the Project goals were undermined by two shortcomings of an otherwise well-conceived project design. In retrospect, in relation to peer education, project planners were over-optimistic that there would be naturally occurring 'communities' of homogeneous identity groups (such as particular groups of sex workers or young people) in Summertown, which could be used as the basis for peer education efforts. It did not adequately anticipate the difficulties that would arise in promoting and sustaining bonding peer relationships in the divided and impoverished conditions in which some of Summertown's most HIV-vulnerable residents lived and worked. Such difficulties would be particularly acute in relation to a project that sought to engage people in fighting a disease shrouded in as much stigma and taboo as HIV/AIDS. They would also be acute in a project involving, among other things, challenging a set of deeply entrenched gender relations. These relations were often tangled up with conditions of poverty and generalized disempowerment in ways that left people with little economic or psychological confidence or flexibility to reshape their life-worlds (particularly their sexual identities) in novel ways. Within such a context, the challenge facing peer education programmes that seek to unite people (such as sex workers or young people), by collective action in pursuit of mutually defined goals in an atmosphere of trust and co-operation, would be a strong one.

The second shortcoming in project design that emerges was the way in which the project planners were over-optimistic and somewhat simplistic in assuming that diverse stakeholders would be equally committed to participating in partnerships in the interests of supporting the Project's proposed activities. It was also over-optimistic in assuming that more powerful groupings would be motivated to collaborate in projects designed to promote the interests of marginalized constituencies with little social power or influence,[43] or to collaborate with non-traditional partners in developing innovative approaches to health, HIV-prevention and the strengthening of the local community to respond to the epidemic.

Within this framework, the remainder of the book tells the stories of the Project's attempts to promote the two participatory HIV-prevention strategies of peer education and stakeholder partnerships in a complex and highly divided community. The first story focuses on sexual health and peer education among sex workers, and the second on sexual health and peer education among young people in school. The third is the story of the Project's attempts to facilitate stakeholder partnerships, including its failure to draw mineworkers into its collaborative participatory framework. While each of these stories is interesting in its own right, not one of them can be fully understood independently of the other. In this sense, these interlocking stories are offered as part of the ongoing challenge of unpacking the frequently made rhetorical claim that health is a social issue, and illustrating some of the complex ways in which the biological, psychological and social are intertwined in ways that cannot be ignored by those who seek to understand health and fight disease.

# II

**Mobilizing Sex Workers to Prevent HIV**
Promoting Peer Education in an Informal Setting

# 4

**Selling Sex**
**in the Time**
**of AIDS**

Sexuality &
HIV-Transmission
among Sex Workers

In the all-male context of the mines, a thriving female commercial sex industry has sprung up. Unskilled and uneducated women in the rural areas of South Africa and the surrounding countries have few opportunities for employment. The possibilities of making a living through peasant farming have declined rapidly and, as a result, women are often totally dependent on their menfolk to support them and their children. When these men are also unemployed, or when relationships with men break down for one reason or another, sex work may be one of the few survival options available.

Part II of this book reports on interviews with sex workers in Summertown, living in geographically isolated shack settlements, housing on average 400 to 500 people, in conditions of extreme poverty, in a hundred or so makeshift shacks. The goals of these interviews were threefold: firstly, to describe the social context of commercial sex in these settlements (Chapter 4); secondly, to give an account of efforts to promote peer education for HIV-prevention among sex workers (Chapter 5); and thirdly, to highlight the limitations of peer education as a strategy of challenging these social determinants of sexuality, in the absence of the support of more powerful local, national and international constituencies (Chapter 6).

Most of the residents of these shack settlements are female sex workers. Others include landladies or landlords (who sell liquor, and provide free lodging to sex workers who attract clients for their liquor businesses) and the *amaHumusha* (unemployed men who make their living on the fringes of the sex and liquor business). The settlements are located near the boundary fences of the mine, within walking distance of mine hostels.

Living conditions in the shack settlements are basic, consisting of windowless tin shacks with no running water or sanitation, located alongside dusty pathways of hard red mud. Both the condition of the houses and the clothes of the people who live in them bear witness to the severity of the poverty that characterizes their lives. Water is carried from a single tap some distance away, and the bush around the settlement serves as an open communal lavatory.

From early in the morning the first customers (miners who have just completed their night shift) come and go in a steady stream to buy sex and alcohol, so that throughout the day the community vibrates with the noise of blaring music and shouting.

Although sex work is officially illegal in South Africa, the authorities have long turned a blind eye on a profession that must have played a key role in sustaining migrant labour and the all-male hostel system.[1] This chapter is based on interviews conducted with sex workers just before the initiation of the Summertown HIV-prevention Project. The aim of the interviews was to provide a detailed account of the social organization of commercial sex work, in order to understand why levels of condom use were so low before the Project's inception, and to highlight factors likely to promote or hinder the success of the programme. These interviews were the first of four sets of annual interviews conducted with sex workers in Summertown, as part of a longitudinal study of sex worker participation in the Summertown Project.

## Informants' life histories

In women's accounts of how they had become sex workers, a number of common themes emerged, including the death of spouses or parents, dropping out of school after falling pregnant, and finding it difficult to find work, leaving an abusive man, or 'running away' from the poverty and hardships of home.

P (19 years old), whose father had died in a mine accident 13 years previously, and whose mother had died of a stroke six years later, had been forced to leave school when there was no money for school fees. After her parents' deaths she and her two sisters had been taken in by an aunt, who eked out an existence on a small income as an informal sector hawker. After a time, her elder sister had gone into commercial sex work. Luckily, a client had fallen in love with the sister (a hope cherished by virtually all the women interviewed). He had told her to give up her sex work and now supported her. After numerous unsuccessful attempts to find a job, at the age of 17 P had been 'recruited' to sex work by an older woman on the mines who had felt sorry for her. P had no sexual experience and her first sexual encounter was a commercial one. In the interview the major concern she expressed was to raise money for school fees for her 9-year-old sister so that she would not be forced into this work. 'Perhaps if all goes well we can help this child to grow up properly.' She was one of only two of the 21 informants who was saving any money, and she was the only one who was open with her family about her profession. She retained a close relationship with her aunt and her sisters, who visited her frequently, and were all aware of her job. Her attitude towards the clients was one of gratitude. 'I respect my clients because they understand our problems, and give us their support.'

M (22 years old) had left school at the age of 14 after becoming pregnant. The fathers of each of her two children had both denied paternity and disappeared, leaving her with a distrustful attitude towards men. Herself the sixth of 11 children, and born in a remote rural area, she had grown up with a violent father who had often beaten his wife and his children (M revealed deep and criss-crossing scars on her back from these beatings). Her second and final pregnancy coincided with her father's abandonment of the family to take up with another woman. Her mother tried to support the family through domestic work, but she had died of a stroke three years previously. After her mother's death M had done 'piece work' in the maize fields at home, but her earnings were too meagre to support herself and two children. Leaving the children with her brother and sisters, she had come to Johannesburg two years previously to seek work, and drifted into sex work when she was unable to find anything else. She had not contacted her family since her departure and said they probably thought she was dead. She felt increasingly disinclined to contact them: first, she said the period of separation made her feel increasingly remote from her old life; second, she felt ashamed to return home without money and clothes for the children (which she could not afford); and third, because of embarrassment they would find out she was involved in commercial sex work. Her attitude to the clients was functional and contemptuous. She said that her only concern was to make money, and she derived no sexual pleasure or companionship from her contacts with them, emphasizing that she would rather live on her own than take the risk of trusting another man.

Several women had run away from physically abusive men. X had run away from her husband after he had broken both her arms. N, badly scarred on her neck, chest and arms, had been severely burned after her former boyfriend had tried to murder her during an argument, locking her in his shack, pouring petrol on it and setting it alight.

J (38 years old) said she had 'run away' from home because she could not stand the hardships and poverty of rural life. She had three years of schooling, having had to leave school after her mother died and her father took up with a stepmother who did not like her. She remained unemployed in rural Lesotho for many years, and had four children. Fed up with the poverty and responsibility, she left the children with her now elderly father and said she was going to Johannesburg to find work. She had not seen her father or children for several years, and said she did not have any money to send to them. Her father frequently sent her messages through relatives. 'He says I must go home to take care of my children. But I can't afford to go and stay with them. I don't know how I would make a living there. I refuse to go back because I don't want to suffer as they all do back home.'

L said she had been lured to Johannesburg by a friend who painted a picture of plentiful money and beautiful clothes. Trapped in a bad relationship in an impoverished rural area with a man who drank too much, she left her three children with her mother and husband to come to Johannesburg in search of a better life. She had also had no contact with her family in the seven years since her departure.

One after another the women told stories of violence, fear and suffering of varying forms. The only exception to this pattern was G, aged 22, who said that she came from a middle-class happy family in a Johannesburg township (where both her parents had been school teachers). She said that she had been a rebel since her early teens, drinking and sleeping around, and had run away from home, impatient with her strict father's ineffectual efforts to discipline her.

The women's life histories suggested that their early experiences had often been characterized by economic deprivation, as well as various forms of physical and psychological abuse, often at the hands of men. In many respects such conditions had not been conducive to the development of a sense of confidence in their ability to take control of their lives or their sexual health. This is particularly the case in relation to insisting on condom use in sexual encounters with reluctant male clients – on whose custom they depend for their survival.

## The organization of sex work

In the interviews particular attention was paid to the form taken by sexual encounters, in the interests of building up a picture of the interactional context within which sex work is negotiated. Women reported between 2 and 18 sexual contacts per week, with condoms used in less than 10 per cent of these encounters. Clients tended to prefer straightforward penetrative sex in the missionary position, the main variation being penetrative vaginal sex from behind. The men usually developed an erection spontaneously while they were negotiating the encounter and before any physical contact. Nearly all the women said that they would not engage in kissing or other foreplay, nor would they indulge in any activity to stimulate a man who did not have a spontaneous erection.

Sexual encounters were initiated in one of four settings. First, there were brief encounters in the open veld beyond the mine fences. During the day, women commonly gathered in groups of four or five and waited to be approached by clients. Clients would generally approach the group and point or beckon to the sex worker of their choice. She would walk up to him, with a fairly typical interaction proceeding as follows:

> Sex worker: Can I help you?
> Client: Can you help me?
> Sex worker: Do you have money? It will be R20 (£2.50).
> Client produces the money and hands it over. Sex worker gives the money to a colleague for safekeeping. Both client and worker move a little distance away, behind bushes if they are available, but often within sight of colleagues if there are no bushes. Sex worker removes her panties and lies down on her back, client takes his trousers down to just above his knees. Penetrative sexual intercourse takes place (usually taking about 3 minutes). Thereafter they both stand up, dress and the client walks away. Verbal communication, apart from the initial negotiation of money, is rare.

It was important to have a colleague standing by, given that a man might pull out a knife after the encounter and demand the money back, or that unemployed men might lie in wait to attack and rob the couple during sexual intercourse.

Similar encounters would take place with men picked up in the mine hostel bars in the evenings or in *shebeens* (informal bars in people's homes) in the squatter camp. Less common were all-night encounters, where a client would pay R50 (£5) to stay overnight with a woman in her shack. There was general consensus that a man who wanted to stay all night was probably missing his wife and family in the rural area, and in need of companionship, as opposed to simply wanting physical release, which would be the case with briefer daytime customers.

There are no pimps, middle men or women involved in the sale of sex. Women negotiate directly with their clients, and keep all of the money for themselves.

Women's accounts of the organization of sexual encounters pointed to sparse opportunities for conversation between sex worker and client, with minimal opportunities for discussion of condom use, except in the case of the less common all-night encounters. However, a range of constraints served to undermine the likelihood of a discussion about condom use even in these all-night encounters, given the elaborate efforts to which women went to model these encounters on non-commercial sexual situations, and to behave as if all-night clients were regular boyfriends.

## Social relationships

Most women in this study were single and led a precarious hand-to-mouth existence, surviving on the proceeds of each day's encounters. Not one was able to give an estimate of her monthly earnings: 'I can't count how much money I make a month – when the money comes in I already have a purpose for it' (M, 22 years old). Few women had much contact with their families of origin or with their own children. Two had no children. The other 19 had a total of 36 children, and two were pregnant at the time of the interviews. Only two of these children lived with their mothers in the squatter settlement. The remainder had been left with family members at home. Most women had left their children in the care of relatives, saying that they were going to Johannesburg to find work, and had simply never returned. At the time of the interviews, four of the 21 women had regular sexual partners (two of these being mineworkers who lived in the hostel and visited on weekends, and two being unemployed men who lived with their girlfriends in the shacks). The criterion for a regular partner was a man who visited regularly and gave the woman an acceptable proportion of his pay packet every month. However, the two women with unemployed boyfriends commented wryly that they, in fact, supported these boyfriends, with one having to pay his gambling debts in addition. Every woman said she would immediately give up sex work if she could find a permanent employed partner.

Apart from the four women with boyfriends, a central narrative shaping the self-presentations was that the women were completely alone in the world, with no support or assistance. However, in the course of the interviews, it became clear that the women did have a range of sources of emotional, material and practical support of varying effect, in particular sex worker colleagues, other community members and, to a very limited extent, some of their clients. Their tendency to say that they had no social support could have been a reference to their relative lack of contact with their family networks, a situation that might be regarded as fairly unconventional in an African context. Half of the informants had had no contact with their families for many years (ranging from three to 15 years), with several presuming that their families thought they were dead. But, despite the lack of contact, these absent families did play a key support role insofar as many of them had taken full responsibility for informants' children, who had often been left behind with the parents or siblings of the sex workers. Some women said that they would have to 'go home' if they became too old or too sick to continue with their work. They hoped that their relatives or children would forgive them for abandoning them and take them in.

*Relationships with colleagues*
While in the interviews women did not emphasize the centrality of their relationships with sex worker colleagues, it was clear that these colleagues constituted a major source of social support – particularly with regard to care during illness, lending money and advice. One of the reasons why women might have underplayed the role of their colleagues in their lives was owing to their ambivalence about identifying themselves as sex workers, and their desire to minimize this aspect of their lives when giving an account of their identities. However, in the course of the interviews it emerged that there is a tremendously strong relationship between the women. Generally working in groups of three or four, they are completely dependent on one another for physical survival in the dangerous conditions of outdoor soliciting, where women were frequently robbed at knifepoint, raped and sometimes murdered.

However, these relationships were not without conflict. Conflicts often arose if one woman perceived that another was taking over her regular clients, or if a newcomer appeared to be attracting a disproportionate amount of interest from the clients. Men were never drawn into these conflicts, and there was an iron-clad rule that men had the right to choose women for sex, and that women had no power to contest these choices. However, once the man had left the scene, his chosen partner might have to endure either verbal or physical assault from her colleagues. Such fights often became vicious when the participants had been drinking. Several women had scars on their faces that had been inflicted in drunken conflicts with colleagues over men. (They referred to the common practice of breaking one's beer bottle and stabbing one's opponent during arguments.)

### Relationships with other community members

On the whole, relationships among shack dwellers appeared to be supportive. Sex workers preferred to bring their clients home rather than servicing them in the veld. If a client should become violent or abusive, other community members could be called upon for protection. However, clients often refused to go to the squatter camp, seeing it as a place where they might be robbed or murdered.

While there appeared to be a high turnover of women coming to and going from the community, there also appeared to be a solid permanent core of 'old women' (women in their 40s). These older women had lived in the community for some time, eventually 'owning' a shack abandoned by a previous woman who had died or left. Within the community, these women were known as people who had been sex workers in their youth, and had given up their work when they got older in favour of the more respectable profession of selling liquor. They also derived respectability from the fact that they 'owned' the shack in which they lived. Owning a shack was associated with independence and control over one's life. As one sex worker put it: 'It is the old ladies that own our shacks who make the rules; we have no control over how we live.' However, informants confided that most of these women still engaged in commercial sex, but did so discreetly. Given their status in the community, no one ever referred to this.

These older women often acted as support figures for the younger women – consoling them, advising them and keeping money for them on the rare occasions when they had money left over after meeting their subsistence needs. (None of the informants had a bank account.) They also presided over savings clubs or drinking clubs composed of groups of women who would meet at each other's shacks.

Women often spoke of the unemployed men who lived in the community. A few of these were also shack owners, and made a living from selling alcohol. Others squatted in other people's shacks and spent their days hanging around, drinking and making their living from petty crime, often stealing money from miners who visited the community. Despite the fact that fear of these men was increasingly deterring miners from coming there to buy sex and alcohol, the interview participants seemed very tolerant of them. These men appeared to constitute some sort of support system for the sex workers, and in particular provided some protection against potentially violent clients.

### Relationships with clients

In the briefer sexual encounters, sex workers tended to have minimal contact with clients. Most commercial encounters were one-offs with strangers. However, friendships of a sort might develop between clients and sex workers who frequented particular bars or *shebeens*, and clients might visit a particular sex worker on more than one occasion.

All but two of the women cherished the hope of forming a permanent liaison with a mineworker, who would agree to support her so that she could give up sex work. Such a man would have a wife and children in his rural area of origin, but he would establish a second home in a shack with a girlfriend. Apart from being a 'meal ticket', a male partner was also an instant source of social status.

> D: In the mine areas, a single woman can only be respectable if she is known to have had a husband or boyfriend who died or left her. Those who have never had a man do not get any respect. In this squatter community if you are single it's even worse – since the only way we survive is through sex. If you are a single woman here, everyone will draw conclusions about your work no matter how discreet you try to be. The only way to be respected here is to have a man.

Against the backdrop of this important economic and social goal, the borderline between business on the one hand, and pleasure or emotional involvement on the other, was often a blurred one. While a few women adamantly insisted that they got no pleasure from commercial encounters, most said they did derive sexual pleasure from some contacts, and that this pleasure was sometimes linked to emotional attachments to clients. In a context where the best economic option for a woman was to find a regular partner to support her, sex workers were vulnerable to the false promises of unscrupulous men. Many ruefully referred to having wasted a lot of time and money through sleeping with a man 'for free'. They would do so on the understanding that a relationship would develop, only to find that at the end of the month he disappeared rather than giving her a proportion of his wages, which would have been the sign that he was a regular boyfriend.

The issue of trust emerged again and again in discussing relationships with men. The overall consensus was that the men were seldom trustworthy. Women frequently spoke of the heartache of these disappointments.

> Q: Before getting emotionally involved with a man, one needs to get to know him first. At month-end he could simply take his pay packet home to his family, without giving you any money before he goes. Men like to be with many women – they just use them and then often they leave.
> Interviewer: But many women do have long-standing relationships.
> Q: Those are women who can stand the heat in the kitchen – even if it hurts them to see what they have to see.

D, six months pregnant, badly burned on her legs from having recently fallen onto a fire, cried through most of the interview. Short of breath and walking with difficulty, she spoke of the stress of having to sell sex in the wet veld to men who showed little consideration for her condition. She had been let down by a miner who had fallen in love with her, told her to give up sex work and given her regular money for almost six months, only to disappear shortly after she told him she was pregnant. She referred to the time with him as the happiest months of her life. She spoke of the pride she had felt in the community status she had had for that short period of time as a woman with a man. Thus, for example, to reflect her elevated status as a woman with a man, during this period of time people had greeted her as 'Sister D' rather than just 'D'. She spoke of the contempt and scorn some community members poured on her now that she had been abandoned.

> D: Life around here is not enjoyable; life around here revolves around jealousy. When I was staying with this man I had everything. He cared for me, supported me. I gave up selling sex and settled down, and people around here didn't understand how I had managed to get a boyfriend. When he left after I became pregnant I was forced to take up the job again, and now it's like people in the community are punishing me, taking revenge. When I suffer from nausea they gossip and sneer at me, telling me that sex workers are not baby-makers, and that we did not come to the mines to make babies.

In short, while there was evidence of strong networks of social support, these were tempered by the jealousies and competitiveness of negotiating survival in a hostile environment where the key resources of survival (clients and boyfriends) were in short supply.

If the presence of social support is an important factor in motivating health-related behaviours such as condom use, the implications of the interviews for the likelihood of successful condom promotion are ambiguous.

## Factors making sex workers particularly vulnerable to HIV/AIDS

What makes sex workers particularly vulnerable to HIV infection, within the context of the way in which sex work is organized and of the support systems available to women? The first factor was client reluctance to use condoms.

In the interviews, women were all well aware of the dangers of HIV/AIDS and said they would prefer to use condoms for every encounter. Clients almost always refused to use them, however, saying that they preferred 'flesh-to-flesh' sex for their pleasure and their health. The principle of selling sex was that 'the customer is always right'. If a man refused to use a condom, the woman dropped the subject and the transaction continued without it. If a woman got too insistent about condom use, the man would take his business elsewhere. Against the background of client reluctance, many women expressed the view that it would be more appropriate to direct HIV-prevention activities at the miners rather than at the sex workers.

> G: If you could work with the mineworkers, telling them about all these diseases, how dangerous they are, perhaps they might agree to use condoms. The decision to use condoms comes from them, not from us. We don't have the power to enforce such decisions.

A second factor undermining the likelihood of condom use was lack of unity among sex workers. In the course of the interviews, women were asked whether they thought an HIV-intervention might have any impact on the community. About a third gave a tentative 'yes', saying that the fact that so many women had agreed to participate in these interviews was proof of an interest in the HIV project, which they regarded as a good starting point.

A key theme running through all their responses was that in order for a pro-condom campaign to be successful there would have to be a degree of co-operation and unity among the sex workers in enforcing it. With the client demand for unprotected sex, unless the women presented a united front, clients would simply take their business to those women who were less committed to sustaining the campaign. Most women felt that the possibility of such unity was unlikely in the face of the chronic shortage of clients relative to the number of sex workers.

C, who had worked for a spell as a sex worker in the Hillbrow suburb of Johannesburg, ascribed the lack of unity to the lack of ambition of her colleagues in the squatter settlement. She compared her colleagues to the far more ambitious and motivated sex workers in the city centre:

> C: In Hillbrow they are serious about making money, they don't have time for drinking. The sex workers here are equally interested in money and alcohol, and this is where the problem starts. People in this community have no interest in uplifting themselves.

D referred to the 'different mentalities' of people in the community. In particular, she highlighted the divisive effects of the poverty and working and living conditions that characterized her community:

> D: People here think differently from one another, they do their own thing, and mind their own interests. If you make a suggestion, some will interpret it in one way, others in another way. Poverty has created a mentality such that some cannot accept it when another person progresses. They want to see us all remaining at the same low level. If you suggest activities to improve people's lives, rather than seeing you as a person being progressive, they think that you are showing off, trying to make out that you are better than they are.

A sense of empowerment, or what psychologists refer to as perceived self-efficacy, is a key ingredient in any successful sexual health-promotion programme. Women's confidence in asserting their right to insist on condom use cannot be divorced from a more general sense of confidence in themselves. Attention to people's life histories pointed to many factors that were likely to have minimized their sense of themselves as confident and valuable. Women tended to refer to themselves as hapless victims of poverty and oppression. Underlying these references, however, was a latent sense of confidence and independence that could provide a valuable resource for community-based sexual health interventions.

Attitudes to their work represented a kaleidoscope of complex responses. On the whole, they hated it and cited numerous reasons why:

> B: The thing I hate about this job is the psychological injuries we sustain. Sometimes you sleep with a person, not knowing if he washes or not. He might have lice, or when you get up you find you have pains in your womb – because the client has drunken herbs for purging which spread diseases. Some people want to touch you everywhere, and do all sorts of things to you. Others talk roughly to you, saying 'Open your legs, bitch'. Eventually such things wear you down. If it were not for the desperation and poverty I would not be doing this.

Every woman without exception said that the work was unpleasant.

> Y: It is a difficult job because it makes us into scraps. We grow old; we get diseases, too many diseases. I look different from when I first came here. My skin has got darker. I am losing weight. I used to have a full body, and I am no longer fresh. In this industry many young women are dying. You see them getting thinner and thinner, and before you can count to three you hear that they have died. Our lives are at risk, but we just do this because of the problems that we have.

Most women said that such diseases were unavoidable, and that there was nothing they could do about them. People referred again and again to the hazards of their work. These included the risk of sexually transmitted infections (STIs) and the loss of reputation, evidenced in the insults and lack of respect with which they were frequently treated. Apart from such concrete disadvantages, there were a few vague references to the fact that the job was 'simply wrong'.

> V: I do get affected psychologically by this work. All I can hope is that God will forgive me, because I really have no alternative. Selling your body is not a good thing, it is simply not right.

They also referred to physical wear and tear.

> A: Often one feels pains during sex. Most of the customers have sex with you roughly. Some of them have very large penises. Even if you try and ask the person not to be rough he will ignore you – he will just tell you that he has paid his money – and go on until he is finished.

The notions of 'respect' and 'respectability' form the cornerstone of African social relations. The respectability of women is associated with the roles of wife, mother and homemaker, as well as behaviours reflecting sexual fidelity and sobriety. In taking on the identity of sex worker, living as single independent women, often with minimal contact with their families and children, informants were separated from many of the markers of conventional dignity and respectability. Engagement in frequent sex with multiple partners, unrestrained use of alcohol and involvement in physical violence were factors that placed them outside socially defined, dignified womanhood. Informants were clear that by doing this work they had downgraded themselves socially and morally.

Women referred to a range of ways in which the community they lived in made it difficult to practise codes of respect. Thus, for example, F defined the squatter community as a place where there were no criteria for distinguishing between right and wrong.

> F: There is a lot of respect at home where I grew up. Here there is no one to guide you on the right path. Even when someone does wrong, no one will say it is wrong. They will say it is right even when it is wrong. Even if you injure someone badly, that will be seen as all right. It's only the police when they come who will say that something is wrong. The people here would defend you, saying, 'You were not wrong, it served them right that you injured them.' Truly there is no respect here.

Sex workers in this case study regarded themselves as 'spoiled' or 'shamed' by their work. Women frequently referred to the job in terms such as 'disgrace' and 'embarrassment'. They said that even children treated them with contempt, a particularly telling sign in a context where they believed that children should treat adults with courtesy, obedience and high esteem. They spoke of the humiliation of being taunted and insulted by mineworkers in public places ('they call us whores, bitches and many names for women's private parts'). They commented on the irony of the sexual double standards that made it possible for their own clients to treat them with such contempt.

> U: It is only a woman who is downgraded by sleeping around, not a man. Men will always retain their dignity, but women will lose dignity.

How do people deal with having a spoiled identity, the stigma of a shameful profession? Despite having failed to meet many of the conventional criteria for respect and respectability, women had redefined these criteria in terms that were more appropriate to their particular working and living conditions. Norms for respectful behaviour in the context of sex work revolved around elaborate forms of denial of one's profession by never referring to it directly. In this sense, sex work was literally 'the profession that has no name'. Denial took a range of forms. Women made strenuous attempts to try to ensure that their families at home did not find out what work they were doing. If they had boyfriends, they sold sex only when the boyfriend was out of the house, and boyfriends often colluded in pretending that they did not know that their partner was selling sex.

Women avoided referring to sex directly as much as possible, even among themselves:

> Interviewer: What language do you use with your colleagues when you discuss the sale of sex?
> V: We call it working. If I brought a man over for the night I would say to my friends that I am going to work. We don't ever even talk about selling.

In negotiating sexual encounters, a range of euphemisms could be used and women stressed that a respectful client never referred to sex directly. Thus, for example, a prospective client might approach a woman and tell her that he loved her. She might then retort: 'I have no time for love. Do you have the 20 rands?'[2] He would then hand over the money, and sex would take place with no direct reference to what was going on.

> A: When we sit at the bar waiting for clients we pretend we are not selling. If a man approaches me too openly I act as if I am amazed, and insist that I am not selling. I ask him what makes him think this is the case; I might even pretend not to understand the words he is using.

In the veld, the commercial nature of sex could not be disguised. In interactions with more regular clients, who would visit the squatter *shebeens* for a drink and then have sex during the course of a social evening, women went to elaborate lengths to model the interaction as if it were a non-commercial sexual encounter. Once the man had indicated that he wanted sex through subtle gestures or indirect reference, he would leave separately from her. She would ensure that they did not return together, so that, if she had sex with another man later on, they could behave as if he was the only man she had had that evening. Clearly, these ideal forms of behaviour were often transgressed. However, they were held up as an ideal, and transgressors – clients who openly propositioned a woman in front of her neighbours, or in front of children, or angry neighbours who used a woman's profession as an insult during an argument – generated anger and bitterness.

Beside these elaborate charades, how else did women deal with their spoiled identity? One way was through a series of justificatory discourses. Predominant among these was the discourse of 'having no option'.

> S: I give my clients respect by telling them I don't like doing this job. I tell them I only do it due to poverty.

> W: This is a job that lowers our dignity. We discuss this often, that we should look for other jobs. But the truth is that there are no alternatives.

Virtually every woman said she had been 'tricked' into starting the job. They all spoke of having been recruited by friends, who tempted them away from their rural homes with stories about jobs in Johannesburg, without telling them the nature of the work. They spoke of arriving and initially refusing to sell sex. Eventually they had been forced into it by a combination of hunger and the lack of transport money to return home. One woman said she had been so angry with her friend when she discovered the deception that she had beaten her unconscious with a stick, and had spent three months in prison after her friend laid a charge against her.

In a paper reporting on similar interviews with sex workers in Gambia, the authors use somewhat judgemental language, variously describing sex workers' accounts of their life histories as 'lies', 'fiction' and accounts that 'could not be trusted'.[3] Possibly this was also the case in the Summertown study. People's stories of being tricked into sex work were remarkably similar. It is speculated that women came to the mines with the primary aim of finding male partners to support them, while realizing full well that they would have to sell sex to support themselves during their pursuit of this quest.

In relation to sexual health-promotion among this group, however, the objective veracity of their accounts is not the most interesting or key feature of the life histories. What is more important is how people reconstruct and account for their life choices, given that these accounts reflect the social identities that are crucial in shaping sexual behaviour. In this context, the main interest of these stories of origin lies in the role that they play as a strategy of coping with a spoiled identity – the way they are used by women to distance themselves from this stigma in as many ways as possible.

These stories serve a useful role in assisting sex workers to sustain a creatively reworked notion of respect and respectability within the context of this least respectable of professions. (Yet while they perform this positive function in one respect, they serve to reinforce women's accounts of themselves as having no option or as victims of fate. In the context of sexual health-promotion, such accounts feed into the broader sense of low perceived self-efficacy that militates against women's empowerment in negotiating sexual encounters, and against the likelihood of insisting on condom use with reluctant clients.)

Another way in which women distanced themselves from their stigmatized profession was to make frequent reference to leaving the job. They continually referred to their intention to look for alternative work in the future, with domestic work being most frequently mentioned. This was said to have two advantages. First, one was assured of a regular and predictable income. Second, this was a job where one 'worked with one's hands' or 'with one's whole body', rather than just 'with one's genitals'.

Another option frequently mentioned by women was that of going home to their rural areas of origin. However, their accounts of what was preventing them from leaving were often contradictory. Thus, for example, women who had explained in detail how they had been forced to leave home because there was no work on the white farms would then express their intention to go home shortly and work on these farms. Many people said that the only thing that prevented them from going home was that they lacked the money for the transport. Yet the money for transport was often not beyond their grasp. It was probably the case that none of them really intended to go home, but that an emphasis on the temporary nature of the work served as another strategy for distancing themselves from their stigmatized profession.

Several women spoke of their shame at having abandoned their families.

> W: On the whole I am a happy person, but I do worry sometimes about going home .... I wonder if my child is still alive or not.
> Interviewer: Do people at home know where you are?
> W: I don't think they know that I am alive .... I'm ashamed and sad that I'm not a responsible mother.
> Interviewer: What do you mean by this?
> W: That I don't buy food and clothing for the child and I don't visit the child – in these ways I am not responsible.

However, they did not act on these feelings. The metaphor of going home served more as a rhetorical device than as a serious option. J captured the ambiguity around this image in her statement 'I want to go home, but I don't want to go home,' but was unable to explain what she meant by this.

Women did not have happy memories of home. Their home lives had often been sites of deprivation, conflict and abuse. On the one hand, their choice to become sex workers had resulted in the dangers and stresses of their present daily lives. On the other, abandoning their claims to conventional respectability (in coming to the mines, abandoning their children and setting up lives as single women with few responsibilities to anyone except themselves) represented a radical break from the drudgery and restrictions of conventional womanhood.

Buried in the interviews, amid all the talk about their intentions to return home at the first possible moment, their shame at abandoning their children and the indignity of the work was a range of comments reflecting this dichotomy. Some said how they enjoyed the wild, often riotous lifestyle of sex work, where in its good moments life felt like a continuous party. They appreciated the freedom from responsibility and decorum. Y feared she would be quickly bored by the domestic routine of cooking, cleaning and child-care that would have been required of her at home. W said she was at her happiest when drinking at the bar with her friends. P reflected the ambiguity that many women felt about the home identities they had given up in a comment in which she started off by idealizing home as 'a place where one did not have problems', but ended up by saying that she would struggle to cope with its staid routine:

P: When I'm at home I don't have problems. My friends and sisters are always there so I'm always happy. But I'm also scared that I might get drunk and do funny things that might make me argue with other people. At home men have responsibilities to their wives – if a man were to buy alcohol for me his wife would come and argue with me. Here there is no such problem – I don't have to answer questions to anybody.

Furthermore, there were numerous suggestions that the women had developed forms of symbolic resistance to the male desires they depended on for their day-to-day survival. One such strategy was to remain completely passive during the sexual encounter:

B: Some, when they are just about to ejaculate, they ask you to 'shake'. But I make him pay if he wants me to shake, he won't just get me to move without paying for it. If the price is 20 rands I want 10 rands extra if he wants me to move.

Another strategy was to emphasize their complete lack of interest in the clients as people, or to emphasize how personally unattractive they found many of them.

Interviewer: Is there any talk between you and the client after you have negotiated the price?
F: We don't talk. What is there to talk about? This person is not your lover, you don't feel anything for him. You don't even know this person.

W: If a client wants to kiss me I refuse. I tell him to get the job over with – he did not come here to kiss me. Generally I just look to the side while it is happening. With some you can't even breathe because of the smell of alcohol or bad breath. Some have sperms that smell bad.

During their more relaxed moments, women would reclaim some of their power by gossiping among themselves behind the clients' backs, joking hilariously about penis sizes, or peculiar sexual styles, or the amusing grunting or screaming noises different men would make during orgasm. There were also references to the tedious nature of male desire.

D: Men don't have self-control. They are just like animals. You sleep with one now, and then he goes around the comer and sleeps with another woman .... I think it's boring – to have a client arrive and you feel tired and make excuses, yet he keeps on pestering you with R20 in his hand.

Despite its dangers and uncertainties, sex work gives women some independence from patriarchal restrictions and the endless responsibility and drudgery of their more conventional roles in situations of poverty. In certain respects it offers women an unusual degree of independence from male control and from the restrictions of the identities of wife, mother and home-maker. Such a sentiment was expressed directly by only one of the interviewees:

> C: I can say I am happy at the present moment because I know how to make a living. I don't depend on anyone like I used to before, where I used to be shouted at if I had to ask anyone for help. I am happy because there is no one who is questioning me. When I do this job, I don't have to ask anyone for anything – I just work hard, and then I can buy anything I want.
> Interviewer: Would you like to have a boyfriend?
> C: I can't say. I'm no longer used to having a partner any more – I don't think I would manage to have a boyfriend .... Since I'm no longer used to waiting for someone to give me money or to depend on. I'm used to being independent. If I were to find a boyfriend I wouldn't manage to go home as often as I am used to doing. He would want more kids. I would have to stop selling sex – this would interfere with me caring for my family – and I can't stand that.

C, cited above, was an exception in the sample in a number of respects. First, she was younger and better dressed than her colleagues. Unlike them, she had experience of sex within the relatively sophisticated urban context of hotels in the Hillbrow suburb of Johannesburg. Here sex work was practised more openly, for better money and received greater recognition as a profession. Second, she was one of the few women interviewed who saw the job as a way of making money to support her family. She herself was one of the children that had been left with an old grandmother by a sex worker mother shortly after her birth, but had taken great pains as a teenager to track down her mother to her workplace in the study community. It was only because she wanted to live near her mother that she chose to spend only part of her time in Hillbrow and the rest of her time in Summertown. Her life's goal was to save enough money to buy a plot in her rural area of origin and to save money so that her mother could retire from the job and have a dignified old age.

However, despite the fact that she was so atypical of the women interviewed, she was one of the few women who had the confidence and the vocabulary to express what for other women was 'unspeakable'. This was the fact that, for all its dangers and stigma, their profession did offer some advantages. For most informants sex work was the profession with no name, an identity so stigmatized and so spoiled that they often avoided naming their work even to one another. Within this context women lacked the discourse to articulate the fact that, although their work was seen as a departure from the conventional and respectable identities available to women as mothers, wives, family members and home-makers, it did have something to offer women in terms of autonomy and independence.

## Conclusion

These interviews were somewhat contradictory with regard to their implications for the likelihood of increased condom use, in a context where
women lacked both economic and psychological power in relation to
male clients. At one level they suggest that the obstacles to the
achievement of the Project goal of increased condom use are almost overwhelming. Attention has been given to the multiple layers of disadvantage
that sex workers face as stigmatized women in a hierarchically gendered
social order. Their lives are characterized by material poverty and
physical danger, as well as symbolic dangers such as the negative image of
their work, and their related lack of confidence in asserting their interests
in relationships with clients. The interview material provides ample illustration of the powerlessness of women, which is repeatedly referred to in
a large research literature on HIV-transmission in sub-Saharan Africa.[4]

At another level, however, there is evidence that women had
constructed a range of psycho-social resources that served to empower
them in their day-to-day lives, and could form the starting point for a
programme seeking to enhance women's self-confidence in condom
negotiation situations. These included a number of creative coping
strategies, such as their reworking of the concept of respectability within
the constraints of their least respectable of professions, as well as various
forms of symbolic resistance to the male desire that formed the basis of
their work. Although women often referred to themselves as 'completely
alone in the world', and referred to conflict and competition among sex
workers, in many ways bonds among women were notably strong,
serving as a dependable resource in times of trouble or danger. There
were also strong ties between sex workers and other members of the
shack community. These included a number of informal voluntary
groups, such as women's drinking clubs and friendship circles and
rotating credit schemes, which women linked into on the rare occasions
that they had spare money.

Moser[5] argues that rather than portraying people who live in poverty as
helpless victims, there is an urgent need for development workers to
develop a more nuanced and creative account of the resources that may
be available to people despite their poverty. Arguably, the psycho-social
coping strategies and social support networks highlighted in this chapter
could be conceived of as community 'assets' of the type referred to by
Moser. The next chapter reports on the study of peer education
programmes with sex workers in Summertown. One of its goals was to
examine the extent to which these assets might form a starting point for
projects aiming to achieve greater assertiveness and confidence among
sex workers. To what extent does it make sense to talk of such networks
and relationships as assets within the poverty and violence of women's
working and living conditions? There is evidence of some success in
using peer education to promote condom use and to reduce levels of STIs

in equally disadvantaged communities of women in countries such as Zimbabwe, Mozambique, Malawi and Zambia.[6] How could peer educational approaches provide the context for a renegotiation of women's social and sexual identities, in a way that increases their sense of control over their health and enhances their motivation to protect it? At the most obvious level, peer educational approaches empower people through transferring health-related knowledge from the hands of outside experts to those of ordinary people, increasing their perceived sense of control over their health. Sexual health-promotional meetings are conducted by 'peers', members of grassroots communities, who derive respect and recognition for their role in promoting health. Furthermore, such programmes often go hand in hand with the promotion of support associations for single women, which provide varying forms of psycho-social and economic support.[7] Such meetings and initiatives rely heavily on pre-existing networks of support and solidarity among sex workers and other community members of the kind outlined in this chapter.

At a more subtle level, such approaches have indirectly served to promote a more open recognition of sex work as a profession, through encouraging women openly to organize themselves into groups dedicated to protecting their interests in an assertive and public way. This openness has challenged the tendency for women to hide their occupations shamefully, denying the nature of their work in pursuit of some semblance of conventional respectability. Women's willingness to organize openly around work-related sexual health issues (which was not the case before the HIV epidemic) has been spurred on by their growing recognition of the life-and-death implications of HIV/AIDS. Peer educational approaches involve open and often very noisy activities that draw attention to the groups involved in them. Thus, for example, women's groups often compose a song referring to the dangers of AIDS and their determination to fight it. This song is sung at the beginning of their meetings to draw attention to their activities, which are generally held in an open space, in an area chosen for its maximum visibility. In a recent interview about the peer educational programme in a particular community, the following comment was made:

> I have been a sex worker all my life and I have never talked about it. Today I am going to talk about it. It's time we stopped hiding this job of ours, or AIDS will kill us all.

A key reason why people agreed to discuss their stigmatized work so openly in this baseline interview study lay not only in their growing fear about the epidemic (whose impact was only just starting to be felt on a large scale in South Africa at the time of the interviews), but also because, in setting up the interviews, much emphasis was laid on the fact that the interviewers regarded sex work as a profession like any other, and had no desire to criticize or judge anyone for their choice of work.

It has been argued that community-based health projects are most likely to succeed when they identify and tap into already existing community resources and assets.[8] It is speculated that successful peer education groups aiming to promote sexual health among sex workers in southern Africa have succeeded in tapping into a range of hitherto unacknowledged but powerful psycho-social and community-level resources and support networks in communities such as the one in Summertown. Many of these networks and coping resources might not previously have been explicitly acknowledged, given the way in which women have sought to deny their shameful professions and represent themselves as passive and unsupported victims of fate. However, the urgency of the AIDS epidemic is growing, combined with a more general climate of growing assertiveness among women. This has given women in a range of African contexts both the sense of urgency and the confidence to acknowledge a range of hidden strengths and resources in the interests of a more assertive approach to their sexual health. The extent to which the Summertown Project could replicate the successes achieved in some other African contexts is the topic of the following chapter.

Facilitating among Summertown
Community-Led Sex Workers
Peer Education

Community-led approaches offer the greatest likelihood of reaching people in the impoverished and 'hard-to-reach' social groups that are often those with the fewest defences against the HIV epidemic. However, given the destructive impact of poverty on social life, the survival norms and networks that communities evolve to deal with hostile social circumstances do not always serve as the ideal starting points for participatory health projects. Such projects tend to succeed best in situations characterized by strong trusting relationships among community members. Furthermore, given that the root causes of HIV infection among sex workers are almost overwhelmingly shaped by a combination of macrosocial factors, including gender inequalities and poverty, the extent to which the impact of macro-social factors can be ameliorated at the local community level is a controversial issue.

Those who seek to place the onus of responsibility for health-promoting social change on people who, in reality, have very little social power are often accused of victim blaming. However, others are less willing to depict poor people as passive helpless victims of their fate. They argue that poor people often have a strong sense of confidence and agency, and that in ideal conditions this sense of agency can be successfully harnessed by community-level projects, leading to improvements in people's lives. This debate continually reared its head in the Summertown Project's three-year case study of a peer education programme led by sex workers in the deprived, divided and violent setting of a local squatter camp.

## Pre-existing 'social capital'? The context of the programme

The peer education programme was located in a shack settlement of about 500 people, with women living and working in very similar conditions to the settlement described in Chapter 4, and located about half an hour's drive away, also on the perimeter of a mine fence. Again the community consisted mostly of sex workers, whose clients were mineworkers, a smaller number of shack owners (landladies and landlords who made their living selling alcohol to mineworkers from informal home *shebeens*) and a smaller group of unemployed men gaining a living on the fringes of the sex and liquor industry. The peer education programme was co-ordinated by the Community Outreach Co-ordinator of the Summertown Project, who was previously a nursing sister in a local health setting and was now employed by the Project NGO. Although she was herself from Summertown, and employed by the Summertown Project, she was external to the small and geographically isolated shack community targeted by the programme in that she was a senior nursing sister with education, wealth and social status beyond the dreams of any member of the shack community. The Outreach Co-ordinator worked with sex workers to establish and sustain the programme. Once the peer educators had been trained, the Outreach Co-ordinator visited the community once or twice a week to monitor peer educational activities and to provide whatever advice and support the peer educator team needed in setting up and running the programme. This particular sex worker peer education programme was one of five similar projects that she set up in similar shack communities in the Summertown region. Part of the Co-ordinator's role was to promote the development of links and networks between these five projects.

The Summertown Project's three-year longitudinal study of this programme took the form of four sets of in-depth interviews with local people (peer educators, other sex workers, and men resident in this particular shack settlement) and with the Outreach Co-ordinator, conducted every year over a three-year period.[1] In this chapter attention is given to interviews conducted six months into the programme.

The geographically isolated nature of the shack community and its informal nature (no formal housing or services) often placed it beyond the influence of the more formal Summertown authorities. Its two links with mainstream Summertown life were the occasional presence of the police when someone was murdered, and the monthly visits of a mobile clinic run by the provincial health department.

Within this informal context, to what extent were pre-existing community networks and relationships on hand to support the programme? Advocates of the concept of social capital emphasize the importance of grassroots participation in local decision-making within a context of egalitarianism and solidarity. In this community, life was full of chaos and danger. High levels of alcohol consumption, poverty and gang conflict made death and injury common occurrences. Despite this, the community was characterized by some degree of organization and discipline, although this cohesion came at a price and was imposed by an unelected 'Committee' of men, referred to in the community as 'gangsters', and led by three 'Chiefs' and their assistants.

The role of the Committee was complex. For example, it ensured safety through community patrols to prevent certain crimes, and through policing and punishment of offenders (whether community members or mineworker customers). Each Monday morning the Committee would organize community cleaning drives to clear up bottles and other litter. It also organized funeral collections to ensure that community members who died would be transported to their place of origin and given a proper burial. Informants regularly cited these burial collections as one of the main advantages of living in the community:

> In other places where there are sex workers, it is bad when they die – because people don't know who they are or where they come from, and there's no one to take care of the remains. Here it is better because we have a custom that you always tell someone where you come from, so that your body can be sent home. And a collection is made when you are dead. (Y, sex worker)

> I am counting on the Chiefs and members of this community to pay for my burial. It's nice to know this because death could knock at your door at any time. They put all the names of the people who are staying in this community in their book. When you die they quickly check if you were someone who contributed to collections when you were alive. If you have been paying for others, we will also pay for you. (B, sex worker)

These funeral collections constituted a key source of community solidarity. As one junior committee member told us:

> We are all staying here as one, and are aware that most of us come from poor families. That's why we had a discussion in the Committee, and decided we should all bury one another. When you have stayed together, known one another for long time, it's a bad situation to think you might be buried by the government. (L, man)

However, the Committee also had a more sinister face. Those who did not immediately produce the funeral money demanded by the Chiefs and their assistants were frequently beaten up with sticks or *sjamboks* (leather whips). Persistent offenders were handcuffed to trees with wire near the main Chief's shack, where they were variously taunted by their enemies and taken pity on by their friends. Eventually someone would come forward to make the payment on behalf of the prisoner in exchange for his or her release. In this respect, the collections were a source of great resentment. Many complained that the punishments were too severe, given that people often did not have the necessary money. Furthermore, many informants felt that they had sometimes been forced to pay for funerals of fictitious people.

> The very same community that protects itself from outsiders sometimes scratches its own people's faces, and I don't like that. The injuries are mostly inflicted by the governors of the community if you don't have money to pay for burials. No one challenges their authority because they are murderers – they are the type of people who just shoot you with no warning. (K, peer educator)

The women interviewed agreed that it was ironic that the Chiefs wielded such absolute power, when women dominated the community both numerically and in terms of their earning power.

> It would be better if women were involved in running the community – the men here rely on us women because we sleep with the miners who give us money. It's us women who support the men here, yet we have no voice on the Committee. [Why don't you suggest to the Committee that they include women?] Yo! They would attack us. (R, peer educator)

When asked why the men had a stranglehold on power, people generally answered, 'It was this way when I arrived here.' Only two interviewees offered a more substantial comment, both in the form of historical anecdotes. A young man offered the first anecdote:

> In the past women were on the Committee, but it was found that they couldn't listen to things, and they used to disagree with other community members. They were indecisive. What is more, there would be relationships between a man and a woman on the Committee, and the couple would defraud Committee money and use it for themselves. (L, man)

An older woman offered the second anecdote. She commented that: 'Not a day goes by without us discussing how we are tired of paying in all this money. We say how we should get together in a large group and confront the Committee about the money they force us to pay them – even for dead people we have never seen.' However, she went on, visibly embarrassed, to tell a story that she said illustrated the 'unreliability' of women, and their inability to act in their best interests.

> Once, we all agreed to defy the Committee at a meeting. Sitting alone as women we were very confident that we should unite in challenging them, but when the actual meeting came only one woman stood up and voiced her defiance, and the rest of us kept quiet. She ended up having to pay a large fine. If we could have stuck together on that issue as women, we would all be living a good life now. Nowadays every time anyone suggests we should call the police when the Committee beats us up, someone refers to that story. Even now we are embarrassed. (S, sex worker)

Both these anecdotes illustrate the deeply ingrained nature of men's resistance to women's leadership, and women's lack of confidence in challenging this resistance.

A second key dimension of allegedly health-enhancing social capital is the existence of relationships of trust among community members. The interviews revealed the lack of trust between women. With complete dependence on mineworkers' custom, the intense competition for clients could lead to jealousy and conflict, often characterized by violence or treachery. While the interviews were being conducted, people spoke of an incident that had happened the previous night. Two women, long-standing friends, were part of a group of very drunk miners and sex workers who were dancing in a local shack at midnight. When one of the women's regular clients started dancing with her friend, she became enraged and stabbed her friend to death with a knife. The police were called, and arriving at about 3am they arrested the woman and hand-cuffed her to the outside of a police van. Leaving their prisoner there, they went into a *shebeen* a little distance away for a drink before returning to the police station. While they were absent, a noisy group of people crowded around the police van taunting the woman, hitting her and stabbing her with safety pins used to keep blankets around peoples' shoulders in cold weather. By the time the police emerged to take her away, the excited crowd had vanished and their prisoner was dead.

Community trust based on a common identity is an important component of social capital. Paradoxically, the common identity that did exist among the sex workers in Summertown was built on extreme poverty and deprivation, and sometimes led to conflict rather than cohesion. When asked, 'what do women in this community have in common?' most women replied 'poverty', which forced them into a loathsome job. Yet it was precisely this poverty that forced women to compete, often viciously, in order to survive. This contradictory situation highlights the complexity of always assuming that common identities constitute community strengths.

In such a context women often rejoiced mercilessly in the misfortune of colleagues. N spoke of the hurt she had suffered after a client had cheated her into giving him free sex by pretending he was in love with her:

> I have learnt not to tell anyone when I am hurt. People laugh at you when you tell them about your problems. Rather than confiding in anyone, in such a situation I refrain from work for two days to sit and think, and after-wards I go back to work. I don't know why they laugh when they too have suffered in this way. Perhaps it's because we don't love one another. Perhaps it's because some of us come from this place and others from that place. And we all compete for men in the business. Perhaps if we all came from the same place we would understand one another better. That is not the case here. (N, sex worker)

Some were doubtful about the possibility of building community soli-darity under such conditions:

> If you have something the others don't have, they hate you for it. Maybe if everyone had the things they needed, it would be better – it's poverty that causes this jealousy. Sometimes we even poison or stab one another to death. (N, sex worker)

Apart from the most serious grievance of selling sex to other women's regular clients, conflicts also arose when people stole from one another;

failed to repay borrowed money; or informed the police against an enemy who might be harbouring stolen goods. When the local 'gangster' band was attacked by 'gangsters' from other areas, this often led to accusations that community residents might have given information to the enemy.

> I don't think people here trust one another. I should never go to anyone for help with my problems. How can you trust a woman who is a drunk, how can one trust a woman who has abandoned her children, and most of all how can one trust a woman who changes men – today this man sleeps at her house, tomorrow a different one. (K, peer educator)

This opinion, from a woman who herself was a sex worker and a heavy drinker, illustrates not only her lack of trust in others but also her own lack of self-respect. There was also a consensus that people motivated by money could not be trusted.

> There is total lack of trust here, because people are only here to make money, so they concentrate on themselves. The reality is that every single one of us only came here for the money, not one person came here for a holiday. (O, man)

A third key dimension of social capital is the existence of relationships of reciprocal help and support. Despite low levels of trust, people referred to numerous instances of reciprocal help and support. These included people lending one another money, particularly for funeral collections; sex workers visiting each other in hospital (taking food or washing the patient in her hospital bed); lending money to women who had recently given birth and were unable to sell sex. Women often referred to other community members as their surrogate families. In particular within-shack relationships often constituted an important source of support, with landlords and landladies often treating their resident sex workers with kindness and generosity.

> We have a good relationship in our house. The landlord buys us food. His wife is like a mother to all of us. (Q, sex worker)

One young man contrasted life in the shack settlement to life in the townships, where he suggested that people had less empathy for those with problems.

> Life here is nicer than the township. Here when you are hungry people do serve you. They say 'we are still cooking but we will call you when we have finished'. In the township, even if they do have food they are stingy – they tell you they do not have food, and tell you to go and find yourself a job. (G, man)

Sex workers often gave one another help and support also, particularly in cases of illness.

> I advised my friend last week. She had an STI and didn't want to go to the doctor. I gave her a bath with Dettol and rubbed her genitals with sulphur. Later when she still had a white discharge I insisted that she go to the doctor, and went with her. (Q, sex worker)

They also offered one another support in the face of exploitative clients. One particular source of complaint was clients who took too long to ejaculate. As discussed previously, most women refused to indulge in foreplay, and clients were expected to develop a spontaneous erection and, ideally, to ejaculate within a maximum of 10 minutes.

> If a client takes longer than 15 minutes, you have to stop him and tell him you want more money. If he does not agree, because he is on top, I push him off and start making a noise to attract my friends outside. When they come in I tell them: 'Hey, this man is mad.' If he still wants to continue he is forced to pay more, otherwise he knows that we will continue to make a lot of noise and embarrass him. (B, sex worker)

(This account, which was given with much laughter, illustrates the humour that many women use as a method for coping with their less-than-ideal life circumstances.)

However, people equally often referred to instances where fellow community members had refused to help. They mentioned cases where shack dwellers with cars would charge extortionate prices to take the seriously ill to hospital, or where the Committee would refuse to lend money to transport a sick person. Many people cited stories of running up to the houses of Committee members to borrow money to transport a sick person.

> The Committee told me to go away – that they only collect money for the dead and not for the living. (S, sex worker)

> People in the community help each other if someone *dies*, they contribute to all the expenses, but when one is *ill*, there is not much support. (K, peer educator)

Unsurprisingly, within such a context, levels of positive community identity and personal morale were low. People's accounts of their lives reflected low levels of self-respect. They characterized the settlement as a community of losers:

> Everyone is here because he or she has failed in life. Failure is the only thing that would drive anyone to a place like this. (M, sex worker)

However, as was the case with women discussed in the previous chapter, there was evidence that sex work, despite its unpleasant aspects, did give women some degree of independence. It freed them from traditional feminine roles in impoverished rural areas, where women often had little power in relationships with men, and where employment opportunities for poor, unskilled, uneducated women were virtually non-existent.

> What I like about this job is that it's an easy way of making money, everything I want I can buy. I do not pay rent and I seldom run out of money like when I was at home. (D, sex worker)

> It's poverty that forces us to humiliate ourselves with this work. But given that we have no choice, it's advantageous as a job – that you can make money without having to shoplift, and risk going to jail. Fashions come and go, you see people dressing nicely and you wish to be like them. (A, peer educator)

The job, for all its indignities, offered economic independence of a sort, and independence from abusive relationships with men.

> I have lived and stayed with men and benefited nothing out of those relationships except for suffering and frustration. As far as I'm concerned it's better to do this work. (B, sex worker)

At the same time, women were realistic about the costs of this freedom.

> We left our families and homes of our own accord. No one chased us away. We left because we wanted to govern and rule ourselves. And now we are compelled to do this job to make a living. Men are tough, sex is painful, they often have large penises that hurt you – some treat you in a dehumanising way, you lose your sense of pride as a woman and as a human being. You are treated like dirt, sometimes that hurts. This is the price we pay for seeking our independence and freedom. (B, sex worker)

In short, the peer education programme was established within a community characterized by conflictual and exploitative relationships, low morale and low levels of pre-existing social capital. Attention is now given to the establishment and reception of the programme, to highlight some of the complexities involved in mobilizing local community networks for health promotion in a community of women whose lives are characterized by multiple layers of disadvantage.

## Building new social capital: The peer education programme

The aims of the programme were to promote condom use, to encourage people to seek early treatment for other sexually transmitted infections (STIs), which increase a person's vulnerability to HIV infection, and to create a climate of tolerance and support for HIV-positive people. This would be done through establishing a peer education network that would provide people with basic information about sexual health risks, distribute condoms and create a supportive context for healthy behaviour. Before the programme condom use was nil. Within a geographically isolated community, where people had limited access to radios, little or no access to televisions, and limited transport money, most people said that before the Project they had known nothing about AIDS and very little about condoms. The Project had played a major role in raising awareness of these issues in the community at large. Furthermore, despite the fact that other STIs have always been a problem in the community, people had little or no knowledge about how to prevent them or treat them.

Women said that they had responded to STIs with a sense of fatalism and powerlessness. They generally 'hoped' they would go away, or relied upon over-the-counter medications (such as aloe vinegar), self-made preparations with herbs from the veld, or the use of douches, drinks or enemas concocted from Jeyes fluid.[2] Medical attention was generally sought only when a woman was unable to walk, by which time she would have to be taken to a hospital in an ambulance. One of the peer education goals was to encourage people to seek medical advice at the early stages of an STI. Virtually every interviewee reported that since the programme had started women had followed this advice, and visits by the ambulance to the community had decreased substantially. The Outreach Co-ordinator had lobbied the local provincial health department to ensure that the free mobile clinic serviced the community more often than had been the case in the past, which made it more convenient for women to seek help with STIs. Before this, the alternative services had been located in Summertown town centre, an expensive taxi ride away.

Another aim of the programme was to increase sex workers' sense of personal vulnerability to HIV as a way of promoting condom use. Biomedical surveys showed that 68 per cent of women were already HIV-positive in 1998 when the programme started. However, cases of AIDS had only recently started to become evident. In the interviews conducted six months after the start of the programme people were in a state of numb fear or denial.

> I haven't seen a person with AIDS, but I have heard rumours that people here have died of it. See – I have lost weight. Perhaps I am infected too. I don't usually use condoms, only with my new clients, but not with my regulars. I do think a lot about the diseases. When I see myself getting thinner I convince myself that it is because I drink too much, or because I am homesick – but there are times when I wonder if I have AIDS or not. We often discuss these things among ourselves, but we usually convince ourselves that our weight loss is due to homesickness. (B, sex worker)

People living with AIDS chose not to disclose the nature of their illnesses to other community members.

I think many people around here are HIV-positive, but are scared to tell others. If it were me, I would not tell anyone around here as they would talk badly about me, and stop my customers from coming to me. If the customers knew I had AIDS they would run away. (N, sex worker)

The fear of scaring off clients was particularly strong since lack of custom meant starvation in a context where there is no social security and no alternative means of support. In addition, interviews bore witness to the stigma and confusion in the community about the extent to which HIV was infectious through non-sexual physical contact or through sharing of cups and plates. This was exacerbated by the fear that one would become a social outcast at the very time when one needed the support and care of one's friends and colleagues. One of the goals of the programme was to work towards creating a climate of tolerance and support that might encourage HIV-positive people to disclose their status.

One starting assumption of the programme was that the likelihood of condom use would be increased through boosting women's confidence in their ability to take control of their sexual health, and through promoting community unity around the goal of trying to increase condom use. At one level, the obstacles standing in the way of these goals were almost overwhelming. However, in interviews conducted six months after the start of the programme, there was some evidence that it was having a degree of impact here. In this regard, the formal aspects of the training of peer educators were only a small component of developing the peer education team. A large amount of additional work had to go into 'preparing' the peer educators for their role, in terms of building both their self-confidence to take on structured responsibilities and their team skills. At this level, the setting up of the programme involved the Outreach Co-ordinator in a series of related tasks.

Initiation of the programme involved a lengthy and sensitive process of consultation with the Committee or 'Chiefs' (*Barena*). They served as community 'gatekeepers', and access to the community would not have been possible without their permission. In gaining this access, the Outreach Co-ordinator had to adopt the norm of approaching the 'Chiefs' with exaggerated gestures of humility and respect, reassuring them that she and the programme would not breach their authority. Once she had gained access to the community, she initiated discussions with sex workers about the possible terms and focus of the project over a number of weekly meetings. Her main goal was to establish a sense of community ownership of the programme.

Peer educators were local sex workers, who were selected through a two-stage process. Firstly, local sex workers nominated a short-list of about 25 women that they believed were most suitable to run the programme. Thereafter the Outreach Co-ordinator selected 15 of these women to constitute the peer educator team, in the light of her opinion as to who showed the most appropriate leadership skills for the work to be done. The peer educators were trained according to the 10-module PSG model outlined in Chapter 2. This included education about STIs and HIV/AIDS as well as training in the use of participatory educational methods, such as songs and role-plays. It also included training in how to set up and monitor a programme. In addition to this formal training, it was necessary for the Outreach Co-ordinator to devote a lot of energy to the peer educators' personal and collective development, in a context where they had little experience of participation in a structured programme, or of working co-operatively towards shared goals.

A key dimension of this work has involved promoting discipline and self-respect. Much effort has been put into working with sex workers to generate their own code of conduct around issues such as punctuality, personal hygiene, dressing appropriately for meetings (e.g. no night-dresses), drinking as little as possible before and during meetings. Another important team-building dimension has been the promotion of conflict resolution skills among peer educators – who told us that, at times, the team has been plagued with conflict, jealousy and gossip. As time passed, the Outreach Co-ordinator was also drawn into other aspects of community life, including the organization and conduct of funeral arrangements for deceased peer educators. She also mediated in the occasional disputes that occurred involving the police, inhabitants of the squatter settlements and the owners of the land on which they were squatting; and organizing black refuse bags to assist people with community cleaning on Monday mornings.

## Community response to the programme

After six months it was clear that the programme had a high profile in the community, and had generated a great deal of attention and controversy. Responses had ranged from unalloyed approval to a more complex mix of scepticism and jealousy of the peer educators. Virtually every informant praised the personal qualities of the Outreach Co-ordinator.

> We needed this programme. It has made a big impact on us. When Sister Z came she showed us all these diseases, and explained them patiently in the style of language that is best understood by us lay people. In the past, the nurses at the clinic outpatients didn't explain things thoroughly, and while some treated us with respect, others were very rude, passing insulting remarks about our profession and looking down on us. Sister Z explains everything clearly and we feel free to ask if there's something we don't understand or any thing we want clarified about HIV or STIs. She is open and kind, she is the best thing we have ever had in this community. (D, sex worker)

The tremendous impact the programme has had on the confidence of peer educators was repeatedly evident.

> I know something good is going to come to me out of this Project – I have made it my life. (C, peer educator)

> Until this Project came here I always felt that I was dirty, that I was nothing. I can't put my finger on what has happened to me since, but I just know that my life has changed. I feel that through this Project I will get my self-respect back. (A, peer educator)

Again and again peer educators spoke of the personal development they had experienced through their involvement.

> I myself am shy, but when the time comes to address a meeting to the whole community I do so freely and without fear that I will not be able to express myself. (K, peer educator)

This sense of pride and achievement had spread to some community members beyond the peer educator team:

> When Sister Z comes in her car, wearing nice clothes, and brings us pens and books, it does give us all a sense of pride. (J, sex worker)

> The peer educators are hard workers, and every time they meet you they will stop and teach you about AIDS. Initially we regarded this as a game people were playing, but now people do listen to them. (S, sex worker)

Some thought the peer educators were working hard and doing a good job. However, others were jealous of the status they received, and even more of the monthly R200 (GB £20) payment they received for their work.[3]

> People think that the peer educators are doing real work, and this is where the jealousy comes in. The difference is that the rest of us get money from using our bodies – the peer educators get theirs through using their brains. (T, sex worker)

This jealousy caused some women to refuse to attend peer education meetings out of spite.

> When the whistle is blown calling us to the meetings, I say to myself 'it's the peer educators who should attend, because they are getting paid, and I am not'. If we go to meetings it will seem as if we are part of the Project, this will contribute to its success – yet at the end of the month they will brag and show us their pay envelopes, while the rest of us have nothing to show for our involvement. (B, sex worker)

The more jealous community members dismissively insisted that the peer educators were motivated only by money, that they did as little work as possible, and that if Sister Z were to withdraw, the programme would fall flat. They also spitefully reported how, despite creating an impression of unity to the Co-ordinator and the researchers, as soon as their backs were turned, the peer educators were known to behave as badly as anyone else, despite their allegedly responsible social positions.

> Not all the peer educators are equally good. Some like to gamble, while others work extremely diligently. When Sister Z is around they are a united group. But when she is not here when they visit one another it happens that some are not working, but rather drinking and playing cards. The whole community is aware of this problem. The programme has not created unity in this community. It will only be done once the peer educators accept that it's up to them to set an example of unity. (O, man)

In the interviews, some interviewees whispered that peer educators cheated on the progress sheets that they returned to the Outreach Co-ordinator (recording the number of meetings and the number of condoms distributed). Others whispered that no one should believe anyone who alleged that condom use was widespread as a result of the programme's efforts.

> People in this community pretend that they are using condoms. Even the peer educators themselves don't use condoms. It's all a pretence to outsiders. They pretend to Sister Z that they are using condoms – yet one of them was recently taken to hospital with an infection. How can you have an infection in your vagina if you use condoms? (Q, sex worker)

Several men argued that the fact that the programme was run by women meant it had no chance of succeeding.

> You see it's like this, where there is no man, there is no unity. These ladies, as soon as you leave, they go back and continue with what they will always be doing. They lose interest and gamble and drink, and the Project is doomed to failure. Things go wrong because of the fact that the Committee was not put in charge of this programme – you have to understand that in this place women only respect men, they do not respect one another. (L, man, junior Committee member)

Women informants varied in their views on the extent to which women were capable of being effective leaders. Two quotes illustrate the disparity:

> In my generation there is a new dispensation altogether. We are allowed to tell men what to do, what we like and what we don't like. (D, sex worker)

> We live in a man's world. It's the men who have to agree on things first, and then we follow. This is the way God created us to be. (S, sex worker)

When asked about community reactions to the programme, people's responses reflected the degree of controversy and attention the programme had generated. Some distinguished between the responses of the uneducated and those who had been to school, between younger and older members of the community, between drinkers and non-drinkers. Others distinguished responses according to personality traits: the 'stubborn' and the 'open-minded', the 'proud' and the 'humble', the 'rude' and the 'respectful'. Older women were reported to be particularly negative, attending meetings only to heckle. Others were said to have responded to talk about AIDS with fatalism.

> When we talk about AIDS, the older women tell us: 'We have been having sex without condoms for a long time and we never died, what you are telling us is nonsense.' (N, sex worker)

> 'Don't waste our time with your AIDS story,' the older women say. 'We are just surviving here from day to day, waiting for the day they have to make our funeral collection.' (T, sex worker)

Landladies and men often refused to lower their dignity by taking an interest in the programme, which they associated with sex workers, the lowest stratum of society. 'What is there that we can learn from whores?' had become their frequent comment.

> Some people are annoyed with Sister Z coming here. These are mostly the older woman, those who are untidy and drink heavily. Mostly from the rural areas. Although such types come from the urban areas also. In fact, those who look after themselves in this community are just very few. (T, sex worker)

And one peer educator commented:

> I think if the peer educators were men people would listen more.[4] You see us women, we began by selling sex, and now we think we can teach them something – we are never taken seriously. They think of us as rubbish, as '*tikilines*' – an insult for a woman who doesn't have a home and who goes around the mines sleeping with every man she meets. But it's only the men who disrespect us. Women are more tolerant. We understand one another's problems, that we do this work because of poverty. (R, peer educator)

Another frequently mentioned fault-line that differentiates responses was that of women as opposed to men.

> It's women who take up the fight against HIV more than men. Because even when we explain about HIV in a meeting with both men and women gathered, you'll see and feel that a woman is more moved and more touched by this than the man. (K, peer educator)

Accounts of the level of condom use varied. Peer educators, concerned about creating a good impression, insisted that condom use was increasing beyond 50 or 60 per cent of women. Others were less optimistic:

> Possibly two or three out of every 10 women use condoms, because customers are scarce and we all have many expenses. Women know that if they refuse flesh-to-flesh they will quickly become broke. Often we are forced to do it, knowing that if I refuse, someone next door will take the customer's money. I try to take care of my life, but sometimes I am forced by circumstances to take a risk. (N, sex worker)

> Sometimes when I really don't have money, when a client approaches me and insists on unprotected sex, I sleep with him without the condom and take the money. I do worry about getting AIDS but this is what I do. (D, sex worker)

These interviews made it clear that the programme had been effective in placing the issue of sexual health and HIV on the public agenda in the community. One of the starting assumptions about the dynamic underlying successful peer education is that collective debate and argument serve as a precondition for the development of new norms. In this respect, in the first six months the programme had succeeded in harnessing community divisions to generate energy and debate around the issue of sexual health and condom use.

## Working with existing community networks as a health-promotion strategy

In line with the philosophy of participatory health promotion, the Outreach Co-ordinator strove to work through and respect existing community structures, and encouraged the peer education team to develop its own norms and approaches for ensuring condom use. However, this could not have been done without the permission of the Committee, which controlled access to the physical space of the community as well as to the sex workers who came to constitute the peer education team and its target audience. Through a delicate process of consultation, the Committee supported the programme, giving the Co-ordinator free and safe access to what would otherwise have been a dangerous and inaccessible workplace.

This support and access was gained partly by giving the Committee a stake in the Project, despite the fact that the sex workers led it. Project funds were paid to the Committee leader to assist the Project by transporting peer educators in his minibus when needed, for example, to enable peer educators to visit other sex worker communities in the region and assist them in setting up similar programmes. Furthermore, Committee members voluntarily took on the role of moving from shack to shack, blowing their whistles to call sex workers to peer education meetings (in the same way as they call community members to their own meetings).

A situation in which it is necessary to collaborate with a violent and exploitative group of armed men in a programme aiming to empower women is contradictory. It highlights some of the dilemmas implicit in trying to follow the directive by health promotion and development agencies that health workers should use existing indigenous sources of social capital as the basis for their work. While such directives may make theoretical and intuitive sense, the task of implementing them in the real world of this programme has highlighted the complexities of working in a context where community networks are structured around unequal and exploitative social relations. The Outreach Co-ordinator dealt with this complexity by often reiterating her respect for the Committee's authority, while at the same time working to demarcate the specific area of sexual health as 'women's business'. In negotiating with the Committee she managed to reach agreement that this is an area in which men had neither the interest nor the ability to play the leadership role that they played in other areas of women's lives. Committee members accepted this demarcation. In other words, they conceded that the limited area of women's sexual health was one that they as men could not understand, and was thus most appropriately guided by the leadership of women.

Some sex workers were positive about the Committee's role in the programme, but others were sceptical about their involvement. Their accounts suggested that the Committee had 'colonized' the programme in a way that fitted in with their autocratic and violent leadership style.

> If you don't want to go to meeting, they will drag you there, and if you still refuse, they will beat you. (J, sex worker)

Some saw the programme as nothing more than a new excuse for the Committee to exploit the sex workers.

> The Committee forces us to attend the peer educators' meetings, saying that those who don't attend the meeting must pay fine of R20 (£2). (V, sex worker)

> The crooks (i.e. the Committee) support the Project for their own benefit and safety – so that we don't infect them with diseases. We are forced to sleep with them because they are Committee members and are in authority. Sometimes we do so willingly in the hope that when the next funeral collection comes we won't be forced to pay. (B, sex worker)

Ironically, however, even those most opposed to the Committee's involvement in the programme still espoused methods of programme management that drew on norms of surveillance or the threat or reality of violent punishment. A key aim of participatory peer education is to increase levels of personal empowerment among target audience members, and improve levels of community trust by creating a context that is supportive of such empowerment processes.

However, not one informant suggested that other sex workers could be trusted to use condoms out of solidarity, or out of having made a public commitment to do so.

> If people don't use condoms, we beat them up, and threaten to take them to the Committee. (K, peer educator)

> If we discover a woman has not used a condom when we are selling in the veld, we demand that she hands over the R20 (£2) the client has paid her, and we give her a few slaps. (J, sex worker)

> If a woman is sick with an STI we encourage the Committee not to allow others to help with money for the doctor. (P, peer educator)

In the interviews, attempts to generate discussion about the possibility of developing non-coercive methods of reinforcing condom use yielded further suggestions involving surveillance rather than being based on trust and co-operation.

> We need to have a system where women check on one another. They should follow each sex worker, and after she is finished with the client, she should be forced to produce a used condom. If she cannot do so, we should write down her name, and report her to Sister Z – and among ourselves we should reach a community-wide agreement that such a person will never be helped by anyone in the community any more. (J, sex worker)

> We should make women put their used condoms in a box, and take it in turns to police the box. This will also serve as a warning to each of us – when a man has an STI his sperms will be yellow. Forcing each one of us to take turns in checking the contents of each and every condom will make us aware of how many of these men might have infected us. (B, sex worker)

The reliance on surveillance at best and punishment at worst – rather than trust – as a means of ensuring programme success is consonant with the methods that local people have developed for regulating their lives in this highly deprived and violent context. Levels of trust were low and the threat of punishment (through public censure, fines or physical violence) was a key means of maintaining community organization.

Do such methods have the potential for promoting a hostile climate within which people with STIs or AIDS will continue to feel reluctant to disclose their status? Or are they a key step towards the creation of new community norms that will result in increased condom use? The interviews highlight the complexity of seeking to locate health programmes within existing local community norms. As stated earlier, community health projects rest on the assumption that community-led health promotional initiatives should, wherever possible, be contextualized within local norms and practices, and resonate with local life worlds. This is believed to increase the likelihood that local people will identify with programme goals, and will assume a sense of 'ownership' of and responsibility for the problem at hand.

While this directive makes excellent theoretical and intuitive sense, the Summertown experience points to the complexity of implementing it in real-life situations. In this setting, local norms and practices were shaped by the struggle for survival in harsh and conflict-ridden circumstances. A setting in which one's physical survival may depend on bitter, sometimes even violent, competition with one's peers was not always the ideal background for a peer education programme that assumed that one was likely to be tolerant and supportive of the difficulties of others in implementing programme goals. Furthermore, the local community networks that constituted this background were enacted within a range of non-local structural inequalities in ways that challenge those seeking to theorize the role of social capital in community development in general, and in sexual health promotion in particular. Much remains to be learned about the extent to which non-local structural and gender inequalities impact on local community efforts to redress problems (such as HIV-transmission) that are significantly shaped by such non-local inequalities.

Writers in the social capital tradition have taken account of the potentially negative effects of local community networks through the concept of 'anti-social capital'.[5] They argue that while local networks and norms might be sometimes be beneficial in their social effects, others may be negative, and still others may be ambiguously positive or negative from one context to another. The Summertown evidence certainly supports this claim. There is a great deal of room for further theoretical development of the notion of social capital in a way that throws light on the processes and mechanisms by which local community networks may have their varying beneficial effects. There is often a tendency to speak of social capital and anti-social capital rather descriptively, as if these positive or negative qualities were in some way the inherent properties of the small local groups. This study suggests that many of these positive or negative qualities cannot be understood at the local level, but need to be understood within the context of broader economic and gender relationships. It is these relationships that frame and structure the nature of small local groups such as this peer education network, in ways that may undermine the best-intentioned efforts to mobilize these networks for positive social gain.

# 6

**Factors Shaping
the Success of Sex Worker
Peer Education** in an Informal Setting

To what extent can community mobilization contribute to the fight against HIV/AIDS in extremely deprived communities? This issue frames a discussion of the possibilities and limitations of the sex worker peer education programme. In many respects, the programme was the prime achievement of the Summertown Project. Although the Project had some success in promoting and co-ordinating biomedical treatment of sexually transmitted infections (STIs), this work was able to draw on existing biomedical infrastructure as well as well-established conventional biomedical frameworks for the conceptualization of health promotion. By contrast, the sex worker peer education programme succeeded in mobilizing strong and confident teams of sex worker peer educators in chaotic and disorganized community contexts with no pre-existing social organization of this nature. It was located in a community with high levels of violence and alcohol abuse, run by women with no previous experience of working in organized and goal-directed teams, and with no local infrastructure to support such work. Furthermore, as discussed later, the context of this work was a larger Project in which, despite a formal commitment to community ideals in the proposal, most of the stakeholders came from a biomedically oriented background. This group of 'experts' tended to be unfamiliar with psycho-social and community-level perspectives on health and health promotion, frequently dismissing peer education as 'vague social science' and suggesting that STI treatment was the only way forward to address the HIV epidemic.

Within this unpromising context, the sex worker peer education programme succeeded in raising high levels of community awareness of the risk of HIV and the importance of condom use in a community that previously had little or no knowledge of HIV. It also succeeded in instilling high levels of perceived vulnerability to HIV, motivating women to seek early treatment for other STIs and distributing large numbers of condoms. To what extent were these condoms used, however?

## Out of the pocket and onto the penis?

One of the challenges facing HIV-prevention workers is not only to distribute condoms, but also to ensure that they are taken 'out of the pocket and onto the penis'. Before the peer education programme, condom use by sex workers was nil. After the first six months, informal estimates by interview participants suggested that two out of ten women were using condoms in some sexual encounters, but not all.

*Eighteen months later*
In the interviews conducted after 18 months of the Project, women estimated that five to seven out of ten women used condoms 'some of the time' in commercial sexual encounters. There was no condom use with regular, non-paying sexual partners. Compared with the patchy levels of interest and scepticism about the Project six months after its inception, by this stage almost everyone interviewed regarded condom use in a positive light, and emphasized its value to the community. There was widespread recognition of the positive role of the peer educators. Not one person expressed jealousy about the salary they were earning. When people were asked if they were jealous, they answered in the negative, expressing their appreciation of the hard work the peer educators did, often for long hours. Several people said that initially they had not taken the programme seriously, and thought of it as a passing fad. However, the fact that it had continued for such a long time convinced them of its worth and of the integrity of both the Summertown Project as a whole, and the local peer educators in particular.

Levels of sex workers' perceived vulnerability to HIV were much higher. There was now widespread awareness of the causes and effects of HIV/AIDS and of the role of condoms in preventing it, as well as a widespread sense of the personal dangers of HIV among sex workers.

The increased credibility of the programme, as well as increased levels of perceived personal risk, was accompanied by growing pressure from peer sex workers to use condoms. While there was general acceptance that some clients simply refused to use condoms, women who did not make a great effort to try to persuade them to do so tended to hide this fact from their peers. Sex workers said that, in the cases when lapses of this nature became public knowledge, women would be chastised by colleagues, and the 'offender' would feel ashamed and embarrassed.

This increase in the local credibility of the Project coincided with a series of events that led to the disbanding of the old self-elected and abusive male Committee. The 'gangster' Chief was murdered by unknown people in a complex series of killings, and the other 'gangsters' either were imprisoned or fled. The old Chief was replaced by a young man in his late 20s who had long resented the absolute power that the gangsters wielded over the community. As leader his policy was to encourage democratic governance of the community, and elections were held for a new Committee, which included a number of women members. This formal recognition of the need for women to be represented may have reinforced the growing respect for the women-led peer education programme in the community.

This complex series of incidents highlights the ways in which the programme often became embroiled in local community dynamics in unintentional and unpredictable ways. Two examples are cited here. The first relates to local suspicions that the Chief's murder was linked to the role he had played in the Summertown Project. As part of an attempt to encourage 'gatekeeper' support of the Project, and as part of a more general attempt to employ local grassroots people as much as possible for project tasks, the Project had employed the Chief to transport the peer educators around in his minibus. Transport was often required when peer educators attended meetings or training sessions at the Summertown Project office (half an hour's drive away), or in sex worker communities elsewhere in the area. As the Project expanded, the provision of transport had become a fairly lucrative source of income. In a community where formal and respectable employment opportunities were few, other men in the community, who also had suitable vehicles, allegedly became jealous that all the work was being given to the Chief rather than being shared out among the men in the community. After his death it was rumoured that the Chief had been murdered by a resident who wanted his job, and very shortly after his death such a person did indeed approach the Project offering to take up his job. (By this time, external Project workers had taken a decision not to employ local people as drivers.)

A second, closely linked incident in which the Project inadvertently became embroiled related to the process of 'changing of the guard' to the new Committee – after the Chief's death and the collapse of the original Committee. For the first 12 months of its existence, the peer education programme was led by a sex worker called 'P'. P was also the girlfriend of a member of the old gangster Committee. She had to flee the community with her boyfriend shortly after the murder of the Chief and two other gang members, for two reasons. First, an unknown person tried to implicate her in one of the murders by burying boxes of Summertown Project condoms in a shallow grave with one of the murdered bodies, which caused much tension among the peer education team. The shooting of a second peer educator, 'L', exacerbated this situation. L was the girlfriend of the man who became the new Chief after the banishment of the old gangster Committee. Rumours developed that L's partner (the new leader) had been involved in the murder of the original leader. In an attempted revenge attack on her boyfriend, L was shot and injured, allegedly by P's boyfriend. The degree of bad feeling set up by this incident within the peer educator team cannot be overestimated.

This incident highlights how projects can unintentionally become embroiled in unpredictable and dangerous situations. In a heavily armed community, characterized by excessive physical violence and alcohol use as well as crippling poverty, events may often move very swiftly in unexpected directions and with unintended consequences. Over the weeks during which this series of events was being played out, trusted local contacts advised the Project's Outreach Co-ordinator that her life would be at risk if she visited the community. The peer education project survived these tensions, however, and grew in strength. In the absence of the Outreach Co-ordinator, and with the disappearance of P (the original peer education team leader), a new leader was elected who remains in place very effectively at the time of writing.

*Thirty months later*
After 30 months of the Project, the achievement of reported condom use by five to seven women 'some of the time' with some paying clients, but still not with regular, non-paying sexual partners, had been sustained. This represented a 'levelling off' of Project achievement in the first 18 months, with no increase in condom use in the year that followed. This is undoubtedly a significant achievement starting from a baseline of no condom use at all. However, patchy condom use in a community where HIV is so rife is at best a partial achievement, given that it is only through consistent condom use that HIV-transmission could be avoided.

## Multi-level determinants of programme success

A range of multi-level factors had an impact on the likelihood of programme success. Some factors relate narrowly to technical aspects of the programme itself, particularly the shortcomings in the way in which the peer education programme was designed, implemented and managed. Other factors relate to the location of this particular peer education project within the broader context of the other Summertown Project activities and to shortcomings of the overall stakeholder management process. These include issues of stakeholder commitment and what is loosely referred to as the extent of stakeholder 'political will' to develop innovative and collaborative approaches to public health promotion. Still other factors relate to internal community dynamics, and to the way in which the strategies and identities that local people had developed to deal with more immediate and short-term threats than HIV/AIDS (such as hunger or violence) were often at odds with Project goals. This point is linked to the more general view that, in situations of poverty and violence, there is only so much that community-level programmes can achieve within broader structural constraints. The research repeatedly points to the impact of non-local structural problems such as poverty, gender inequalities and migrant labour on the transmission of HIV, and on efforts to prevent it. The findings re-emphasize the importance of fighting HIV at three levels: the short term (the biomedical control of STIs), the medium term (community-level peer education and condom distribution) and the long term (large-scale national efforts to reduce poverty and empower women).

## Poverty as a major obstacle to programme success

The link between HIV and poverty is frequently emphasized by those who seek to discredit the value of community-level approaches. This link is an undeniable one, and is nowhere clearer than in this sex worker peer education programme. However, armchair commentators (usually in universities in more affluent countries) often criticize those who advocate community-level approaches to HIV-prevention as 'victim blaming', through placing responsibility for social change on communities who are in fact the victims of economic inequalities beyond their control. Such critics often advocate strategies such as the global redistribution of wealth as the only solution to the epidemic. Such throwaway blanket statements are intellectually lazy, and often serve as an excuse for inaction. They are intellectually lazy because their generalizations about links between large macro-social processes, on the one hand, and micro-processes such as sexual intimacy, on the other, are sweeping. Such generalizations fail to provide any account of the factors that mediate between these two levels of analysis, in the interests of beginning to tease out how and where multi-level social change programmes should best devote their energies. They lead to despair and hopelessness because sweeping analyses of this nature do not have immediately actionable implications for those facing the enormity of the death and suffering that exist at the coal-face of the epidemic in deprived communities.

They also fail to take account of the fact that, while many participatory grassroots projects have indeed had disappointing results, there are also many examples of successful community projects, where marginalized women have succeeded in improving their lives, and even in contributing to the possibility of more lasting social change. Such improvements are often on a scale that seems small to more affluent outsiders in the West, but are tremendously significant in the lives of the women concerned. African feminists resist western feminists' tendency to depict African women as passive victims of inexorable social forces. Such 'victimological' language is seen as deeply conservative insofar as it perpetuates conceptual frameworks that freeze marginalized women into passive social roles, obscuring the possibility that small-scale collective action might have the potential to feed into multi-level movements towards social change. It also ignores the possibility that, while not having access to material resources, poor people still have other strengths and other assets that they can – under some circumstances – mobilize to their advantage.

The grassroots community group who played an important role in initiating the larger Summertown programme (of which the sex worker peer education programme forms one component) did so because they believed that a community-level intervention would be useful. This group included representatives of township teachers, religious ministers, youth leaders, unemployed people, sex workers, traditional healers and local politicians. Most of these people would have had extremely unpleasant first-hand experiences of life in the apartheid era, with all its violations and indignities, as well as representing large numbers of people living in poverty today. When this grassroots group approached a number of epidemiologists, social scientists and community workers, and asked them to assist them in setting up a community-led HIV-prevention programme (after their earlier grassroots efforts to find funding for such a programme had been unsuccessful), there were two options. The first was to work with this group to set up the programme, involving, for example, putting them in touch with international project funders, working together to write fundable proposals, and assisting in implementing state-of-the-art biomedical and community development methods (which have had some – albeit patchy – successes in reducing STIs and HIV in particular countries and contexts). The second was to inform grassroots community members that their collectively negotiated and carefully thought-through desire to set up a community-led HIV-prevention programme was a waste of time, based on an inadequate understanding of Africa's problems. On this basis, one might have advised them to put their energies into fighting poverty and countering the effects of global capitalism. The Summertown Project resulted from taking the former option.

Having said this, however, the Summertown experience repeatedly highlighted how poverty facilitated HIV-transmission, as well as undermining prevention efforts. With the benefit of hindsight, could some of the obstacles to programme success have been addressed in principle, even in the absence of parallel poverty-reduction programmes? Much work remains to be done in developing understandings of the processes and mechanisms by which poverty undermines the social fabric of communities, leading to the transmission of disease and hindering HIV-prevention efforts. Within this context, one of the goals of this book is to highlight how poverty and gender inequalities shape and constrain community dynamics in ways that serve to undermine local efforts to improve people's health. Given the key role of community-led participatory approaches in efforts to combat HIV all over the world, there is certainly room for far more explicit and detailed debate and argument about the possibilities and limitations of such approaches.

## Mechanics of programme design and implementation

*Programme variation, materials and support*
Starting with a narrow focus on technical issues of programme design and implementation, as time passed attendance at weekly peer education meetings dropped. At the most superficial level, the technical challenge of sustaining people's interest and motivation to attend weekly meetings over a three-year period was a strong one. People got bored with the repetitive content of the meetings, complaining that they recycled the same old STI information again and again. Where possible, the Project's Outreach Co-ordinator tried to supplement the Project's educational

material with information about other health problems, such as breast cancer or tuberculosis. However, the task of providing ongoing materials of interest is a resource-intensive one that could not always be sustained by a lone community worker with a huge workload and no access to project materials or technical support. (A breakdown in communication meant that the Summertown Project's anticipated relationship with a Zimbabwean-based peer support group was not sustainable.)

Furthermore, while peer educators were trained in a range of participatory educational methods (dramas and role-plays, for example), with the passing of time they slipped back into the easier, old-fashioned didactic teaching styles that are known to have limited impact. A pattern developed over time whereby, unless the Project's Outreach Co-ordinator or outside visitors were present, peer educators would simply lecture the audience with charts depicting various STIs. In the first two years, while the Project's Outreach Co-ordinator was actively involved in the programme on a weekly basis, she was present to inject enthusiasm and confidence into the peer educator team. In the third year, in line with the Project's goals of 'community sustainability', and because of the need to initiate new peer education projects in new sectors of the community, she was encouraged to play a less active role in the programme. As her profile increasingly lowered, the programme lost a degree of status and credibility. As she withdrew, it became clear how much her high-profile presence had served as a draw to meetings. Without it, attendance at meetings declined considerably.

A third reason for the drop in attendance was that, somewhat ironically, people said that the new and more democratic leadership style of the new Committee meant that people were no longer coerced into attending meetings. There was less external pressure to attend than had been the case when the gangsters had blown their whistles calling women to meetings, and threatened or punished those who did not want to attend.

The goal of achieving 'local sustainability' of community projects in chaotic and impoverished communities may be an over-optimistic one. Participatory peer education is often mooted as a method of choice because it is inexpensive to implement. This is a misconception. Participatory approaches are needed because they take the best account of the psycho-social and community-level determinants of sexuality. However, the task of ensuring survival of peer education programmes in 'hard-to-reach' communities requires a great deal of effort and energy.

The problems resulting from the Outreach Co-ordinator's gradual withdrawal highlighted how much her personal charisma and status had enhanced the effectiveness of the Project. AIDS activist Mkhondzeni Gumede argues that that it is vitally important that HIV/AIDS programmes select staff who have 'passion' and commitment.[1] Sustained passion and commitment by project workers is necessary to continue to motivate action in groups of people, such as the sex worker group in this Project, who may have had little or no experience of engaging in collectively empowering activities.

*Economic empowerment programmes?*
In relation to the topic of programme variation and advancement, a great deal has been written about the need to supplement peer education programmes of this nature with economic empowerment programmes for women. It is argued that, since poverty is the major obstacle to condom use, with sex workers' survival depending on condom-averse male clients, condom promotion programmes that do not provide sex workers with a means of supplementing their incomes are unlikely to succeed. Against this background, the Outreach Co-ordinator worked hard to motivate women to look into the possibility of developing alternative income-generating schemes. In response to discussions about possible ventures, women suggested child-care crèches and vegetable stalls. One group of sex workers started selling vegetables from a stall in the area, but gave up after two weeks. They said that it was boring and relatively unprofitable to sit all day in the hot sun in the hope that their equally impoverished co-residents would patronize their small businesses.

Other women showed little interest in attempting similar enterprises. Some had developed a highly mobile lifestyle, moving from one area to another. Some moved in response to changes in the availability of clients from one area to another. Others moved in response to their belief that clients tended to patronize 'new faces'. Others were continually on the move owing to anxiety about their precarious immigration status. Such women were reluctant to establish income-generating schemes that would involve putting down roots in one particular area. Others argued that the local area was already saturated with small businesses, and that existing shack residents had already exploited existing commercial opportunities to their utmost limit. Others saw mainstream income-generating activities as unrewarding drudgery in comparison with sex work which, for all its disadvantages, yielded financial rewards that were not only immediate, but also far in excess of what could be raised in a small business.

Against the background of this lack of interest, the Project's Outreach Co-ordinator decided that her energies would be better spent working towards the development of a healthier and safer culture of sex work than working to encourage a few individual women to develop income-generating projects. This was due not only to the lack of interest among sex workers in the development of such projects, but also to her perception that, even if such projects were to succeed among a small group of women, there would always be a steady stream of poorer women coming in to fill their places. The continued existence of the sex work industry appeared inevitable in a national and regional context characterized by high levels of rural poverty and lack of unemployment opportunities for unskilled women, and it was beyond the means of a small local project to take on challenges of this nature.

*The development of critical thinking*
Freire emphasizes the development of critical consciousness as a central component of the development of empowerment, and as an important

precondition for behaviour change.[2] Thus a key component of critical consciousness is an understanding of the way in which one's behaviour is structured by broader social and structural forces. Among sex workers, this might include the development of a critical and self-conscious analysis of the way in which gender relations and poverty impact negatively on people's sexual health. It might also include reflection and debate on how women could work together to ameliorate the impact of structural forces on the likelihood of condom use. However, sex workers tended to explain condom use in individual and asocial terms, including a harsh, punitive and unsympathetic view of those who do not use condoms. Rather than contextualizing their judgements of one another within a more critical understanding of the way in which sex workers are victims of social problems (in particular poverty and male oppression), women who did not use condoms were often caricatured as weak or bad individuals. There is an urgent need for the development of peer education materials that provide the context for participants to develop more sociological views of their sexual lives and choices.

The dearth of critical thinking was evident not only in women's punitive and victim-blaming analyses of condom use and non-use, but also in sex workers' reluctance to criticize the peer education programme constructively, in the spirit of collective critical reflection, about ways in which the programme could be improved or restructured in light of particular local conditions and needs. Because people valued the programme so highly, and feared that any criticism of it would lead to its withdrawal, they tended to speak of it in one-dimensional and non-critical ways. In the interviews, the reluctance to criticize the Project was particularly strong among the peer educators and their friends. The opposite trend was observed among those who were not in the peer educators' circle – this group was happy to gossip and criticize, but in a destructive and carping way.

There is much room for the development of materials that promote two interrelated dimensions of critical thinking within participatory HIV-prevention programmes. The first is critical thinking about the social influences on condom use. The second is constructive reflection on the strengths and weaknesses of projects seeking to promote condom use, in ways that enable programmes to grow and improve in line with local conditions and local needs. The intersection of these two forms of critical thinking constitutes a crucial milestone on the road towards the development of critical consciousness of the social obstacles to behaviour change. They also provide the context in which women can collectively examine ways in which they might work to ameliorate the impact of such social factors on their health and well-being.

## HIV programme goals at variance with strategies for coping with poverty and other life challenges

The strategies and identities that local people developed to deal with more immediate and short-term threats than HIV/AIDS (such as hunger or violence) were often at odds with Project goals. For many women, HIV was simply one new link in the chain of life-threatening phenomena that had characterized their lives, and they were slightly puzzled by all the attention that this particular crisis had generated. For some, a virus that began with invisible symptoms – and that would take years to manifest in full-blown AIDS – did not seem as pressing a problem as the day-to-day struggle against poverty and violence.

*Fatalism, denial and stigma*
People had developed a range of psychological coping mechanisms for dealing with the dangerous and bleak working and living conditions that frequently presented them with stressful situations in which they had little power. The first coping mechanism was fatalism. Peer educators said that there was a hard core (up to a third of their potential target group) of what they referred to as 'stubborn' women. These were women who insisted that there was nothing they could do to protect themselves from HIV/AIDS. They said that it was no more or less serious than many other challenges that they had faced in their lives, and that they were unwilling to take too much notice of it. While a sense of fatalism probably serves as an effective coping strategy, enabling women to cope with repeated experiences of threat in dangerous and bleak working conditions – in situations where they have little power or control – it also had the unintended consequence of increasing their vulnerability to HIV/AIDS.

Other coping strategies included those of denial of risk, and stigmatization of people living with HIV or AIDS. The role of defensive denial when dealing with life-threatening risks of all kinds is well-documented.[3] The stigmatization of people living with AIDS, as well as a widespread denial of personal vulnerability, were key obstacles to programme success. Denial and stigma are psychological defences that protect people from what threatens to become an intolerable level of fear and anxiety by leading them to deny that they are at personal risk of overwhelmingly frightening problems. Part of this process involves projecting fears of one's personal vulnerability on to stigmatized out-groups, and in the process dissociating oneself from a sense of personal risk of the feared problem. One particularly well-publicized case of such fear, stigmatization and denial was the stoning to death of township AIDS activist Gugu Dlamini, shortly after she had made a public announcement that she was HIV-positive. Among Summertown sex workers, one of the worst insults one could deliver in a fight or an argument was to 'accuse' someone of being HIV-positive. Almost every person interviewed said that if she was HIV-positive she would never tell anyone for fear of gossip and abuse, as well as fear of rejection, loss of clients and loss of love from regular partners. It is incidents and attitudes such as these that make many people scared to discover their HIV status, or to keep it a secret, even from close family members and neighbours, when they do.

Despite a baseline survey that revealed that 68 per cent of sex workers were HIV-positive, and anecdotal evidence for a string of AIDS deaths, people chose not to disclose their HIV status, and deaths were generally attributed to other causes. Thus people might say: 'She died from drinking too much', or 'He died of tuberculosis'. In the interviews, even in the third year of the Project, people repeatedly said that a key determinant of their lack of motivation to use condoms was a lack of first-hand experience of people who openly acknowledged that they were HIV-positive or had AIDS. In the absence of local people prepared to disclose their status, the Outreach Co-ordinator invited a woman living with AIDS from a nearby township to address the community, in an attempt to persuade sceptics about the existence of HIV. However, most people did not believe she was HIV-positive because 'she looked so well'.

It is increasingly argued that the development of tolerant attitudes, as well as humane and effective systems of care for people with AIDS, should be a key pillar of any prevention strategy. While the Summertown Project was constituted as a project concerned with HIV-prevention rather than AIDS care, any success it might have will go hand in hand with the important complementary role being played by the local 'Home-Based Care' movement in some parts of Summertown. This is a programme that trained local people in elementary nursing skills to enable them to care for people dying of AIDS in a context where hospital facilities and medical assistance are often beyond the capacity of already strained medical services. A key dimension of the struggle against the stigmatization of people with AIDS, and people's denial of personal risk, is the creation of a tolerant and supportive attitude to people living with AIDS. This is a long-term and daunting challenge.

### Alcohol

In a community that makes its living from the sale of sex and alcohol, levels of alcohol consumption are high. People who are drunk are less likely either to remember to use a condom or to be motivated to use one even if they do remember. People repeatedly cited the use of alcohol as a major obstacle to condom use. This was another situation where the goals of the HIV-prevention programme were contrary to a range of economic and psychological survival strategies. Alcohol played a positive role in people's lives in a number of respects. Income from the sale of alcohol was a key component of the community's economic survival. The symbolic link between drinking and womanizing was frequently made in the interviews with mineworkers, for example.

Apart from its economic significance, alcohol also served as a psychological coping mechanism, a form of medication for dealing with the violence, poverty and stress of daily life. It served as an essential component of the loss of inhibition that women felt when proposing sex to men, in a cultural context where women were strongly prohibited from taking the sexual initiative. It was also cited as a source of harmony in what often was otherwise a divided community.

> People here are not close, they are very cruel. The only time we are happy is when we are drunk. Drinking with lots of people makes this community a lovely place to be, we sing and dance. (K, peer educator)

Alcohol was also a source of conflict, violence and stigma. While there was some degree of tolerance for drinking by men, women who drank to excess were often the source of contempt in the community ('just look at her, she is so drunk and dirty, and even carries a beer bottle in the street'). There was a perception that women who drank too much 'could not be trusted'. Alcohol sales to mineworkers served as a source of violent competition, sometimes between *shebeen* owners. It also caused tension between *shebeen* owners and sex workers when the latter ignored the community rule that only shack owners were allowed to sell alcohol (with sex workers surreptitiously trying to sell single bottles of beer to clients in sexual encounters, to keep the profits for themselves).

Whatever the role played by alcohol, people were unanimous that drinking undermined the likelihood of condom use. Some women referred to female condoms as a solution here. If a client was drunk enough, it was often possible for a sex worker to insert a female condom without him noticing. If a sex worker was planning to drink, she said that if a woman put on a female condom a couple of hours before drinking it would mould to the shape of her vagina and remain fairly well-positioned, provided she remembered to move the flap aside when she urinated. However, despite the fact that sex workers frequently expressed a preference for female condoms, these are expensive and currently not distributed as part of any state or non-governmental organization (NGO)-funded HIV-prevention programmes.

In interviews, people were asked what could be done to reduce alcohol-related harm. Suggestions included fining people who drank too much, limiting the opening times of *shebeens*, providing jobs so that people didn't have the time or motivation to drink so much, and installing lights in the community so that people could identify drunks who raped women or robbed mineworkers in the dark. However, these strategies were put forward with scepticism. Some work has been done in Europe on developing community-based alcohol policies that, rather than seeking to promote abstinence, focus specifically on reducing alcohol-related harm.[4] With the role that alcohol plays in undermining sexual health, there is much scope for the development of such policies and approaches in the southern African context.

*Mobility*
Although there was a solid core of permanent residents in the shack settlement of this study, reference has already been made to the highly mobile lifestyles that some women chose. Many were constantly on the move, travelling from one sex worker site to another. Some women moved in response to fluctuating customer demand, driven by factors such as industry retrenchments or the building of new factories employing large numbers of migrant men. Others moved when they felt that local clients were starting to get bored with them. Still others moved when they were drawn into gang fights or community conflicts that placed their lives in danger, and others in response to fears that their families might find out where they were, especially given the efforts that women made to hide the nature of their work from parents, siblings or children whom they might have left behind. Whatever the reason, this high turnover of women, with newcomers generally having little familiarity with condoms or HIV-prevention measures, presented the peer educators with another strong challenge. In interviews, some newer residents were not aware of the programme's existence. Other newcomers said that the profile of the programme was so high that they could not have avoided knowing about it almost immediately. In short, while the programme was doing a good job of reaching some new residents, it did not always link up with others. Furthermore, it appeared that peer educators were sometimes a little hard on newcomers, simply handing them condoms and expecting immediate compliance before they had attended any peer education meetings or had a chance to familiarize themselves with the programme's goals.

## Forgotten constituencies

*Sex workers' non-commercial boyfriends*
An important constituency that was 'forgotten' in programme planning and implementation was that of the sex workers' non-commercial regular boyfriends. These were frequently unemployed or informally employed men living in the squatter settlement. Even among the most HIV-aware and pro-condom sex workers, who tried their best to use condoms with paying clients as much as possible, not one woman attempted to use condoms with her regular, non-commercial, sexual partner. In interviews at the early stages of the Project, women justified this convention through their belief that their boyfriends were at best entirely faithful to them, or at worst used condoms with casual sexual partners but not with them, their regular girlfriends. The unrealistic optimism of this claim emerged when some sex workers participated in a biomedical STI prevention research programme in the shack settlement in the third year of the Project, which involved regular testing for STIs. Participation in this research highlighted how even women who were the most successful in using condoms with clients were frequently reinfected with STIs by their

boyfriends. Detailed discussion of this issue, in the context of these STI findings, led to sex workers acknowledging openly to one another that their boyfriends must be sleeping around without protection. It also led to their acknowledgement that boyfriends, as well as clients, played a key role in the spread of STIs.

However, even though sex workers had acknowledged this to one another, a range of social norms and psychological obstacles prevented a free and frank discussion of STIs with the boyfriends. In the final set of interviews, sex workers were more open about this problem than they had been in earlier interviews, saying that they were powerless to insist on condom use with boyfriends who disliked condoms.

> The man I stay with is always sick. I wanted us to go to the clinic together for HIV testing, but he refused. I went alone, and I was negative. I still worry about HIV though, it's been a long time, and I still doubt the man I stay with. I am just expecting it to happen. But I lost guts to speak to him about condoms since he refused last time. [Would you leave him?] Leaving him is not an option. (J, sex worker)

Boyfriends disliked condoms because they said it diminished their sexual pleasure and also because they wanted children. They were allegedly not co-operative in women's attempts to negotiate condom use.

> I asked once, and he beat me up. (D, sex worker)

> I asked once, and he accused me of not trusting him. (X, sex worker)

The notion of trust within relationships was a complicated one, with women often having to go through elaborate conceptual whirligigs to sustain it.

> You don't trust a client, but you will trust your boyfriend, even if he cheats on you. You trust him because you stay with him. If you get a disease, at least you know where it comes from. (N, sex worker)

As was the case with clients, women often had limited negotiating ability when they were financially dependent on men.

> My boyfriend won't use condoms. He laughs at me when I suggest it and calls it a plastic. I trust him. No, I don't like the idea of sex without condoms, perhaps he has sex with someone besides me, but he's helping me support my children, there's nothing I can do. (I, sex worker)

As discussed earlier, there is a tradition where sex workers often made every effort to hide their work from their boyfriends, who also pretended to be unaware of their girlfriends' profession.

> I am not sure if my girlfriend (of two years) is a sex worker. Once you meet a girlfriend and get involved with her, they don't say much about sex work to you. (P, man)

By the same token, boyfriends made every effort to hide their casual encounters from their girlfriends, who colluded by turning a blind eye to this. It appeared that, symbolically, non-use of condoms was seen as a valued and positive affirmation of trust and faithfulness, and played a key role in maintaining comforting myths of fidelity in a community where there was, in reality, very little fidelity.

The choice of not using condoms with regular boyfriends, as a way of demarcating some relationships as special and valuable in comparison with commercial sex, is another coping strategy that women have developed to deal with their particular life circumstances. Within this context, flesh-to-flesh sex meets a desire for intimacy in a generally hostile environment. There is still a great deal of work to be done in developing understandings of how to promote safe sex in close regular relationships, where partners have very strong unconscious emotional needs for intimacy and trust, symbolized by flesh-to-flesh contact. Such needs might be particularly strong in the high-stress situations in which sex workers live and work. Furthermore, in designing sexual health-promotion programmes for sex workers, much more explicit account needs to be taken of the potential role of non-commercial boyfriends in the spread of disease in sex worker communities.

### 'Respectable' women

As discussed, the Project sought to strengthen two types of community relations, conceptualized as 'bonding' and 'bridging' varieties of social capital. It sought to strengthen community in the narrowest sense, through building *bonding social capital*. This refers to strong and trusting relationships within groups of homogeneous people (for example, sex workers in a particular geographical location). Although the Project succeeded in building a degree of bonding social capital among a group of like-minded sex workers in this shack settlement, this group by no means included all the women living in the community. The peer educators characterized a group of 'stubborn' women who refused to take the programme seriously. The way in which the programme was constituted also discouraged the participation of women who chose to sell sex in a more clandestine manner, as well as married women who were not sex workers.

There is a stigma around sex work, a factor that limited the number of women who were prepared openly to participate in Project activities. A key focus of the Project was to empower sex workers to feel less ashamed of their work, so that they could work assertively and confidently towards improving their occupational sexual health. In this regard, its open sex worker focus was essential. However, this image alienated and excluded a lot of women who sought to hide their professions – married women and older women went to particular lengths to keep their work a secret.

Even outside the context of sex work, there was strong community distaste for the notion that 'older people' might be sexually active. In a community where life expectancy was low, and where heavy drinking and difficult living conditions aged people prematurely, anyone over the age of about 35 was considered an 'older person'. Aside from this general distaste for the idea of elderly sexuality, in a society where age was associated with wisdom and gravitas, older people were expected to set an example for younger people, and were therefore even more stigmatized for engaging in a non-respectable profession. In such a context, older women sold sex in secret and in isolated settings, often without the support networks available to younger sex workers who practised openly and in groups, and who could also participate openly in sexual health-promotion activities. Older women also often had difficulties in attracting clients, and as a result were said to be particularly reluctant to insist on condom use for fear of alienating the clients.

This situation highlights the challenge of designing programmes that simultaneously empower sex workers to be more open about their work, on the one hand, but include opportunities for the participation of women who seek to maintain a more 'respectable' image, on the other. (There is also an urgent need for programmes to find ways of attracting women who are not sex workers, given that many monogamous African women contract HIV from their husbands.)[5] One cannot assume that 'sex workers' are a unitary group who will have equal access to peer education networks.

## Lack of 'bridging' social capital

The Summertown Project was designed in a way that sought to be mindful of the material and the psychological inequalities between sex workers and their mineworker clients in two ways. The first was through the development of a women-focused peer education programme led by sex workers. This would provide women with a context in which they could exercise leadership and control of the programme in a way that would not have been possible had men been involved. Secondly, the Project was designed with full awareness of the frequently voiced criticisms of the limitations of HIV-prevention efforts that target most behavioural change and condom-promotion activities at women, in situations where men hold superior economic and psychological power in the control of the sexual encounter. The Project sought to accommodate this insight through the establishment of parallel peer education programmes among mineworkers, the paying customers in the commercial sex encounter. The intention was that these parallel programmes would be synchronized both in terms of the timing of their implementation and in terms of technical excellence. It was anticipated that there would be some interaction between these peer-education networks – including, for example, 'bar-based meetings', where sex workers and clients would hold joint activities in bars serving alcohol to mineworkers – the bars to which sex workers sometimes went to find clients. However, there was general recognition that such efforts were unlikely to succeed without the development of various forms of bridging social capital – particularly the full participation of the mineworker trade unions, and mine management representatives – in order to ensure the co-ordination of efforts targeted at different constituencies.

A range of obstacles stood in the way of the development of peer education on the mines – and over the three-year period of study most of the mineworkers did not participate in peer educational activities. Condom refusal by mineworker clients continued to be a problem facing the sex worker peer education project throughout its three-year life, testimony to the difficulties of motivating very different interest groups to co-operate around unified HIV-prevention goals in a community as complex as that in Summertown. Key to the success of of community-based HIV-prevention programmes needs to be the development of *bridging social capital*, which is defined in terms of the promotion of relationships between diverse and heterogeneous groups of people who might normally not have had much contact or experience of working together, but whose collaboration is needed to optimize programme success. The health problems of poor communities, such as this small shack settlement, often derive from economic, political and social arrangements that lie beyond their immediate geographical boundaries. The efforts and resources of grassroots communities may be ineffective if they are isolated from the support of those mainstream economic or business groups or political institutions that hold the power to enable or undermine the impact of their efforts.[6] In particular, programme efforts are most likely to succeed in the context of co-operation between local communities and appropriate private and public sector networks and policy-makers.[7]

The Summertown Project failed to build three forms of bridging social capital that would have greatly facilitated the chances of programme success. The first form that would have facilitated the empowerment of sex workers would have been the establishment of a network of links between the Summertown sex workers and similar groups of sex worker peer educators in other parts of southern Africa. A large 'gender and development' literature emphasizes that local women's empowerment programmes should develop links with regional and national networks of similar women, in order, among other things, to increase women's confidence and to build up a critical mass of people working for similar social changes. Collective action should extend beyond local boundaries through the development of channels by means of which the views and needs of grassroots groupings can be articulated to policy-makers at the broadest levels.[8]

The Project was originally to have been part of a southern African peer education network – which includes programmes run by 'women at high risk' in a number of regions and countries in southern Africa. However, following a series of inter-agency breakdowns in communication, the anticipated Summertown participation in this networking process did not materialize. After 18 months an external project evaluator recommended that efforts be made to establish links between sex worker peer education teams in Summertown and regional and national bodies (including self-employed women's unions, and national sex worker organizations concerned with promoting the interests of sex workers). Although the latter bodies do exist, they tend to be small, under-funded and based in large urban centres. Their activities and debates are often dominated by more educated urban sex workers, and their lives and interests may be poles apart from the geographically isolated and severely marginalized and destitute women in Summertown; there is, however, an urgent need for the latter group to be represented on such bodies. However, the Summertown Project's funding proposal had not specifically allocated funding or human resources to facilitate such a networking process, which would have been extremely resource-intensive, given the isolation of this sex worker community, and their total lack of experience of participation in such networks. The Project's Outreach Co-ordinator was unable to facilitate this process, given that her local responsibilities were often well beyond the time and energy of one person.

The second form of bridging social capital that would have facilitated success of the sex worker programme involved the co-operation of the mining industry and trade unions in promoting the development of parallel peer education programmes aimed at mineworkers (originally intended to be part and parcel of the project's proposed 'stakeholder collaboration process'). The lack of mining industry and trade union commitment to building bridging networks in order to promote the success of peer educational efforts was a key obstacle to possible success. A range of institutional obstacles, as well as what will later loosely be referred to as a lack of 'political will' on the part of the mining industry and trade unions, meant that over the three-year period of the study most of the mineworkers were not exposed to peer education.

Although it has continually been emphasized that the 'political will' necessary to fight HIV/AIDs resides not only in the will of formal governments, but also in the will of other groups that shape the economic and symbolic contexts within which HIV flourishes, this does not mean that the formal government does not have a key role to play in shaping the likelihood of success of community development projects. This is the third area where lack of bridging social capital may have undermined the sex workers' efforts. A large development studies literature points to the important role of 'state–society synergy' in successful development projects. Such synergy is said to exist where local community development efforts are backed up by supportive government policies, and by the efforts of public officials who work collaboratively with local community residents to 'co-produce' desired outcomes, such as improved sexual health. Although there was sometimes a degree of synergy between sex worker groupings and provincial government health officials, national government disunity and vacillation over the existence and causes of AIDS undermined the support and solidarity that a small local programme would have derived through being part and parcel of a wider national anti-HIV initiative. These points are taken up in Part IV of this book.

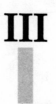

# III

**Mobilizing Young People to Prevent HIV**
Promoting Peer Education in a Formal School Setting

# 7

## 'Condoms are Good, But I Hate Those Things'

Sexuality & HIV-Transmission among Young People

**This chapter was co-authored by Catherine MacPhail**

In this and the next chapter, the focus turns to factors shaping sexuality and the likelihood of peer educational success among young people in Summertown. As stated earlier, over the course of the three-year study, the Summertown Project sought to promote participatory peer education among three groups in Summertown: sex workers, young people and mineworkers. Some of the factors shaping the likelihood of peer educational success in the relatively chaotic and informal setting of the squatter camps in which sex workers lived and worked have been examined in Chapters 4 to 6. A number of the challenges face peer educators in the sex worker context, related to the informal and relatively disorganized setting in which they implemented their project. Intuitively, one might have thought that implementing peer education would be easier in the more institutionalized and organized contexts of the formal school system. Yet, this very institutional setting posed as many constraints as possibilities for peer educator teams. The extent to which some of these constraints can be addressed, and some of these possibilities maximized, is a crucial issue for the health and well-being of millions of young South Africans.

Young people have rocketed to the forefront of HIV/AIDS-prevention campaigns in southern Africa. A growing number of surveys are pointing out that young people between the ages of 15 and 25, especially young women, are particularly vulnerable to HIV infection, with levels of up to 60 per cent in some groups. These figures highlight young people as an obvious group for targeted interventions, insofar as the vast majority of young people under 15 are *not* HIV-positive. This means that young people in their early or mid-teenage years are a promising group for prevention efforts. Furthermore, with the significant number of young people in school, many members of this vulnerable group are located in an already established institutional framework within which HIV-prevention programmes could be implemented.

In this chapter the focus is on the construction of sexuality among young people in Summertown, with reference to the way in which community and social level factors shape the transmission of HIV infection. This is done in the light of one survey study after another that points out that young people often engage in high-risk sex, despite knowing about the dangers of HIV infection. Informing people about health risks is not enough for behaviour change. High-profile leaders and academics at international summits and academic conferences constantly call for more energetic pursuit of programmes of behaviour change as a way to address the epidemic, with particular focus on young people. Yet the understanding of the factors that hinder even the best-intentioned programmes aimed at young people is still in its infancy. This chapter points to some of the factors that militate against behaviour change, drawing on focus groups among young people in Summertown. Chapter 8 presents a case study of a behaviour change programme in a township school, in the interests of highlighting the factors that undermined the programme's well-intentioned attempts to reduce HIV-transmission among school learners.[1]

## The extent of HIV among young people in Summertown

The extent of the epidemic among young people was still not apparent in the mid-1990s when the Summertown Project proposal was formulated. For this reason, this group was not originally a specific focus of the Project, which identified mineworkers and sex workers as the groups living and working in situations that placed them at highest risk. However, a community-wide survey conducted in 1998 pinpointed young people as particularly vulnerable to HIV, despite sound levels of knowledge about sexual health risks. The HIV prevalence was 0.2 per cent for boys and 8 per cent for girls aged 15 and 39 per cent for men and 58 per cent for women aged 25.[2] A second survey conducted exactly one year later, in 1999, showed that the levels among young women had risen in the intervening year, with an HIV prevalence of 2 per cent for boys and 13 per cent for girls aged 15 and 35 per cent for men and 68 per cent for women aged 25.[3]

Why is it that young people are so vulnerable to infection? And why is it that young women are so much more vulnerable than young men? Although much remains to be learned about this, the answer may lie in a complex interaction of biological and social factors. At the biological level, some studies have suggested that male-to-female transmission is more likely for every sex act than the reverse.[4] It has been suggested that male-to-female transmission of HIV for every sex act may be twice as likely as female-to-male transmission if no other sexually transmitted infections (STIs) are present, and four times as likely if either partner has a genital ulcer. Two major biological reasons have been put forward to explain this asymmetry in transmission. First, differences in the genital contact surfaces mean that lesions are more common in women than in men, increasing the likelihood of the exchange of body fluids – the medium of HIV-transmission. Second, in unprotected sex, women are exposed to infectious fluids for longer than men. While men are in contact with body fluids containing the virus just for the duration of the sex act, women remain in contact with semen for much longer. In addition to these biological factors, various social and behavioural factors may be important. There is much still to be learned in this area. Recent studies have pointed to the age differences between partners as one significant determinant of such differences.[5] Young women in Summertown tend to have sexual relationships with men who are, on average, five years older. Given that HIV levels increase with age, this means that young women are at greater risk from older partners than young men are from their younger partners. Another factor relates to the fact that it is not unusual for sexually inexperienced young women to be forced into unwanted sexual encounters, which may increase their biological vulnerability owing to the increased likelihood of female genital damage resulting from forced sex. This might also be one expla-nation for the high levels of HIV infection among young women who have only had one sexual partner.[6]

## Context of condom use by young people in Summertown

As part of the Summertown Project social science research, a series of baseline interviews and focus groups were conducted in order to inves-tigate the social factors that make young people vulnerable to HIV infection, and to understand the context within which HIV-prevention efforts would be located. This research found that young people had high levels of accurate knowledge about the causes of HIV/AIDS and the fact that it was incurable (which remains the case for the vast majority of young people in Summertown, who lack access to the resources for drug treatment). They were also aware of the 'ABC' approach to prevention (Abstain, Be faithful or Condomize). However, a range of factors under-mined the likelihood of condom use. These were: low levels of perceived vulnerability to HIV despite high levels among their peers; peer norms around sexuality and condom use; limited access to condoms; adult disapproval of youth sexuality and condoms; gender inequalities; and economic constraints that impacted on young people's sexuality in a range of complex ways.

### Perceived risk of HIV infection
An important requirement for translating knowledge into behaviour change is a feeling of personal vulnerability to HIV infection. Both locally and internationally, there has been a tendency to characterize HIV/AIDS as a disease of 'others'. This 'othering' serves as a psychological defence, protecting the individual from anxiety through externalization of the

threat on to identifiable out-groups such as homosexuals or commercial sex workers, resulting in a sense of unrealistic optimism about one's own vulnerability. Surveys in Summertown suggested that, despite high levels of infection, 70 per cent of young men and women said that either there was no chance of their becoming infected or they didn't know whether or not they were personally vulnerable.[7] There were conflicting views among young people about the incidence of HIV in their community and the extent to which they and other people in the community were vulnerable to infection. Some felt that HIV and AIDS were not very common. Others felt that the disease was a problem in their community and that personal experience with AIDS had forced people to acknowledge that it really exists. It was more common for young women than men to state that HIV was a problem in their own community. Young men tended to view HIV as a disease associated with atypical behaviours such as rape and commercial sex, or with excessive alcohol consumption. Young men often referred to the risks of being unwittingly infected by a woman who had previously been raped or who had not informed them that she was a sex worker. In such discussions, the implication was always that it was the woman's responsibility to insist on condom use.

> AIDS is spreading because of the prostitutes. You meet a woman and tell her that you want sex and she takes you to her house. Sometimes you are a group of guys and she will sleep with all of you. She will not be thinking of condoms at the time. (Boy, aged 13–16)[8]

Most young men suggested that, if they themselves were to become infected, this would be the result of someone else's actions. Such a person was usually portrayed as a deceiving or irresponsible woman, who would have unprotected sex with them, despite knowing that she was HIV-positive.

### Peer norms around sexuality

Young people's sexual encounters were conducted within the context of a peer value system, in which men were depicted as sexually driven, active and predatory, and young women as largely passive victims of male desire. Young people's talk about the act of sex invariably prioritized the penetration of the vagina by the penis, with an exclusive focus on the achievement of male pleasure. No reference was made to female sexual desire, or to the possibility that women might also experience pleasure from the sexual encounter. Significant adults (parents, nurses and teachers) tend to deny the existence of youth sexuality, choosing to turn a blind eye to any evidence of it. As a result, many young people's sexual relationships are conducted hurriedly and beyond the adult gaze.

Among young women, there was great peer pressure to be seen to have one steady boyfriend, as opposed to young men who came under pressure to be seen to have multiple sexual encounters. Sex was considered an integral part of any relationship, and young men who let their friends know that they had not had sex with a girlfriend were teased and taunted.

> Guys were asking me how I could not have had sex with such a nice girl. They said I was stupid. They said I didn't know anything about sex. That's why any girlfriend that I get, I want to make sure that I have sex with her. (Boy, 13–16)

Peer norms often militated against condom use. Young people may be negative about the contraceptive implication of condoms in contexts where having children provides young men with proof of their masculinity, and gives young women a role in contexts where opportunities to finish school or find valued work are few.[9] Other young people argue that condoms are only worth bothering about if one of the partners is known to have an STI.[10]

While many young people emphasized the importance of using condoms and their intention to use them in relationships, it was clear that peer norms undermined the likelihood of their consistent use. Both young men and women said that condoms were generally unnecessary in 'steady' relationships but that they should be used in casual encounters.

> It's if you have two girlfriends, your 'steady' and your secret lover. You would never use a condom with your 'steady', but you should use one with your secret lover – because you don't know if she has a disease. (Man, 21–25)

Within regular relationships, trust militated against use of condoms. Young women argued particularly strongly that, if a steady partner were to insist on condom use, this would indicate a lack of respect and trust within the relationship.

> If a boy wants to use a condom a girl will say this is because he disrespects her – because he wants to use 'a plastic'. (Girl, 13–16)

Young men known to be using condoms would be jeered at and belittled by their friends. Many said that they had been accused of being 'stupid' after telling peers that they had used condoms, and as a result they had decided that they would not use them again. Young men said that in contexts where young men would often stand by during their friends' sexual encounters to warn of approaching adults, there was little chance of using condoms without being noticed.

Young people, particularly men, made distinctions between sexual contacts requiring condoms and those that did not. Such distinctions were often made on the basis of the partner's appearance or sexual reputation. Trust was also referred to as a key reason for not using condoms.

Such trust was expected to operate unconditionally – with no reference to the discussion of a partner's past sexual history or of asking whether one's partner had had an HIV test.

There was repeated clear evidence of the way in which dominant social norms placed young people's sexual health at risk, and of the way in which the vast majority of young people subscribed to these norms. Young people in this study did not, however, constitute a completely homogeneous group in terms of their sexual behaviour, nor were they incapable of reflecting critically on their own actions. This is a particularly important precondition for the success of peer educational approaches, which rely on the stimulation of debate and discussion for the testing of dominant norms and alternative ways of behaving.

Thus, despite stories about the taunting suffered at the hands of peer groups, there were some young people who had chosen not to conform to peer pressure by deciding to postpone their sexual debut. Young men in this category were all members of church groups that forbade sex before marriage. Reference was also made to young men from rural Lesotho who had come to Summertown to find work, and who had chosen to remain celibate owing to strong familial relationships preventing them from engaging in behaviour that would disappoint their parents. A minority of young women also resisted stereotypical notions of females and condom use. One participant in particular said that she enforced the use of condoms in her relationships and that, to ensure condoms were always available, she carried them herself.

> I refuse. I don't want to be doing that without a condom. I can say no thanks. I also think that the best thing is to always have condoms in your pocket because you don't know what time you are going to have sex. (Woman, 17–20)

However, these young people who spoke of resisting peer norms were in a small minority.

### Condom availability

Condoms were available from a number of sources in Summertown, both free from government clinics or from commercial outlets such as shops and social marketing programmes. Despite this, young people still spoke of instances in which they had had unprotected sex because they did not have access to condoms. Difficulties in procuring condoms were particularly acute for young women. First, they referred to the negative attitudes of nursing staff at the local clinics.

> I won't go to the clinics. The nurses shout at you. They get angry when you take condoms and sometimes when you have relatives who are nurses they ask: 'What are you doing with condoms? Do you have a boyfriend? I am going to tell your mother.' (Woman, 21–25)

In many countries and contexts poor people's interactions with state representatives and infrastructure are marred by 'rudeness, humiliation, harassment and stonewalling'.[11] South African hospitals are no exception, with a recent study pointing out that nurse–patient relationships are often characterized by humiliation of patients, and even physical abuse.[12] Experiences of humiliation by nurses were particularly common among young women in this study, many of whom said they no longer went to local clinics after having had unpleasant experiences with clinic staff when seeking advice about their sexual health.

Another factor deterring many young women from using condoms was their fear of getting a bad reputation. They spoke of gossip as a constant source of conflict and stress in the township. They said that a woman who was known to carry condoms risked being labelled as promiscuous or as a 'bitch'. Young men supported these claims, saying that they wouldn't trust young women who carried condoms.

> Yah, it will worry a guy if a girl carries lots of condoms. He will worry that when he's not there, what is she using them for? It means that I'm not alone in having sex with her. (Man, 21–25)

However, some of the older young women said such pressures did not deter them.

> The community says: 'She likes sex because she's carrying a condom in her bag.' I disagree. I think that such a girl is taking care of herself because she doesn't want to be affected by STIs, AIDS and unwanted pregnancy. (Woman, 17–20)

(The above quotation also illustrates the point made above about negative social attitudes to female sexuality.) Some young men agreed that young women carrying condoms did not always indicate that they were 'promiscuous'. This minority of young men agreed that it was important that their female counterparts should protect themselves.

However, most people suggested that carrying condoms indicated that a young woman was 'looking for sex'. This was considered a grave insult and a threat to the good name of a young woman, in a context where there was such great pressure on young women to portray themselves as the passive objects of male desire, and strenuously to resist any suggestion that they might themselves want or enjoy sex. Within this context, young women have a particular investment in portraying any sexual encounters that they engage in as unintended, something that 'just happened', in a way that militates strongly against condom use.

> I don't always have a condom when I need one. Sometimes you don't know when sex is going to happen because he just asks you to come. Then you need a condom and it's not there. (Woman, 17–20)

*Adult views on sex and condoms*

Throughout the discussions there were oblique references to the role that adults inadvertently played in undermining young people's sexual health. They spoke of living in small, inward-looking neighbourhoods where close-knit networks of parents often informed one another of their children's suspected sexual activity in attempts to limit their behaviour. While there is concern among adults about the spread of HIV and STIs among the youth of the township, adults do not condone the use of condoms but prefer to encourage abstinence through punishment and gossip. Indeed, during feedback sessions at the end of research group discussions, many of the participants indicated that this was a rare opportunity to discuss sexuality with an adult who would not punish them, and expressed a desire for their friends and siblings also to have this opportunity.

> The problem is that they just beat you for having sex. Others will just condemn you and spread the rumours around that you misbehave. They don't give you any advice. (Boy, 13–16)

Male participants stated that parents' disapproval of youth sex was often the reason that they didn't use condoms at all. Most lived at home with their families and indicated that their opportunities to have sex were constrained by their parents. When the all too rare opportunity arose, condom use was seen as a waste of the precious time that adults were absent from the home.

Many young people referred to the poor role models set by adults, who gave them mixed messages about sex. On the one hand, they got strong messages that sexual activity was taboo and wrong. On the other hand, they said that after heavy drinking many adults themselves indulged in relatively public sex, which served to contradict the 'sex is taboo' messages put out in other contexts.

*Economic context of adolescent sexuality*

A lot has been written about young women's inability to demand condom use in conditions of poverty, where boyfriends are often considered an important source of economic assistance. When sex is exchanged for gifts, young women's ability to negotiate condom use is said to be limited. Much has been written about the 'Sugar Daddy' phenomenon in other southern African countries, where younger women sleep with older men in exchange for money for school uniforms or other essentials such as soap or transport. Older men are obviously more likely to have paid work to finance such exchanges. In such contexts, however, even unemployed younger men are expected to provide gifts of money or clothes for their sexual partners. Male students in Uganda jokingly refer to young women as 'dentists', humorously suggesting that young women's desire for money would drive them to extract the very gold out of their sexual partner's teeth if they could.

In the Summertown research, a few young men and women portrayed the sexual act as one in which women were motivated by the expectation of lifts home from school, gifts or subsistence cash.

> This school is some distance away. Sometimes the students struggle to get lifts to school. Others will sleep with the guys who give them lifts. (Boy, 13–16).

In sexual exchanges of this nature, women had little power to demand the use of condoms if their partners were unwilling. However, in the Summertown context, relationships of this nature seemed to be the exception rather than the rule. Many young women did indeed expect gifts in the course of their relationships. Furthermore, many young men who were still at school commented ruefully that it was hard to find and keep female partners when one was not earning money. However, most young women did not view relationships primarily as a source of income. The impact of poverty on poor sexual health is often mediated more indirectly through a diffuse array of processes. Research in southern Africa suggests that while, in the early stages of the epidemic, HIV spreads uniformly across all economic and educational levels, at the later stages, people with greater access to money and education are more likely to change their behaviour as a result of HIV-prevention programmes, and hence less likely to become HIV-positive.[13] Research in Mozambique has suggested that schoolgirls from schools in wealthier suburbs tended to report fewer sexual partners, more frequent condom use, expressing a greater willingness to challenge stereotypical gender norms, and reporting far more assertive behaviour in relationships with men than was the case with young women attending schools in poorer suburbs.[14] Adverse economic conditions affect young people's capacity to deal with the threat of sexual ill-health in a range of complex and indirect ways, and not simply through the commercialization of sexual encounters.[15]

*'We don't call it rape, they're our boyfriends': Gendered power relations*
Young women's ability to negotiate the conditions of sexual encounters freely is dramatically limited by the imbalance in power between young men and women in heterosexual relationships. A range of factors constrains their ability to refuse sex or negotiate the use of condoms. In various South African contexts, researchers have pointed to the way in which young women's attempts to discuss condoms or AIDS before a sexual encounter has led to rape or violence.[16] HIV/AIDS and violence against women have been referred to as the 'twin epidemics' facing South Africa.[17] The interviews in this study emphasize the need for much more research into the impact of sexual violence on the high levels of HIV/AIDS experienced by young women in South Africa. In these interviews and focus groups, young men spoke of tricking young women into

having sex, lying about their intentions to use condoms as a way of persuading reluctant women, or forcing women into having sex with groups of their friends. In addition to sexual coercion, there was reference to physical violence, with several young men referring to the practice of punishing young women who had too many sexual partners by beating them, to teach them a lesson. Women suggested that sexual relationships focused around male desire and the satisfaction of male needs and pleasure, with women being relatively powerless to demand relationships on other terms.

> This is because usually men have ninety per cent and women have ten per cent of power. Men are heads of the family so that causes trouble because they can abuse women. (Girl, 13–16)

If sex is not willingly provided, many men in the community feel that they can insist on it as being a necessary part of a relationship and as proof of their girlfriend's love. Violence and coercion are often used on unwilling sexual partners.

> They find you on the street and they force you to go home with them so that they can have sex with you. It is rape but we don't call it rape because they are our boyfriends. (Woman, 21–25)

Counter to the majority practice of male dominance in relationships, there was a small minority of men in the study – all of whom belonged to religious organizations – who heatedly defended the rights of women in sexual relationships.

> There must be an agreement about sex with your girlfriend. There is a problem when people do it forcefully. (Boy, 13–16)

Only one woman spoke of actively resisting male power in coercive situations. She spoke of physically attacking a friend who had tried to force her to have sex with him, causing him to flee in terror. Other participants in this focus group expressed admiration for her courage, saying they would have felt powerless to act in such a situation.

The Summertown research on young people's *first* sexual encounters found that rape or emotional pressure was common, and foreplay was minimal or non-existent. Reference has already been made to young men feeling pressurized by their peers to have early and frequent sex with as many partners as possible. This pressure often translated into a degree of force or coercion of young women in sexual encounters. In a context where young women have few opportunities to learn about sex, it was not unusual for them to report that in their first sexual encounter they had no idea what was happening to them. Many young women remember their first sexual encounter as painful and unpleasant, regretting that it had happened.

*Resistance to stereotypes*

There is a frequently voiced criticism of those social scientists who make generalizations about gender relations and gender identities. Critics argue that generalizations of this nature ignore the array of options available to people in constructing their gender identities. Conscious of these critiques, one of the express goals in the research was to focus specifically on examples of counter-normative behaviour. This goal was formulated not only in the interests of avoiding such criticism, but also because of an interest in peer education. Peer education participants who have counter-normative ideas play a key role in contributing to the processes of debate and argument that drive successful peer education forward. Wherever possible, in presenting the research findings, attention has been given to counter-normative gender identities and behaviours. However, it was apparent that the degree of freedom that young people have to resist social stereotypes may often be constrained in the marginalized settings in which many Summertown youth grow up. Many young people had few role models of counter-normative sexual behaviour and counter-normative gender identities, and their life circumstances were often characterized by a lack of opportunities to develop a critical consciousness of gender relations and alternative ways of being.

## Conclusion

At one level it seems bizarre that a community with such high levels of youth HIV is locked into such a conspiracy of silence around the risks to young people. Young people and their parents persistently cling to attitudes and norms that will lead to high levels of suffering and death. In many ways this is a community that is trapped in high levels of passivity, denial and fatalism about a problem that is likely to kill off half its young people. Parents and clinic staff adhere to old-fashioned views that deny the existence or desirability of teenage sexuality – in the face of massive evidence to the contrary. Young people cling to stereotypical views about gender, trust and relationships that militate against sexual behaviour change, at the same time as knowing about HIV and its risks. However, in the next chapter it will become clearer why these responses are not as strange as they seem. Social and sexual attitudes and norms, and the possibility of changing them, are shaped and constrained by broader contextual factors – which are examined in the following case study of a peer education programme in a township high school. Many lessons remain to be learned about implementing sex education in ways most likely to protect young people from HIV infection.

# 8

**Facilitating** | **among**
**Community-Led** | **Summertown Youth**
**Peer Education**

### This chapter was co-authored
### by Catherine MacPhail

The frequent high-profile calls made at countless international summits for measures to change the behaviour of young people as a key dimension of the fight against HIV-transmission in Africa have been mentioned on several occasions in this book. Yet, in the face of limited understanding of how to change young people's behaviour, these calls have a hollow ring; there is an urgent need for further investigation of the nature of the gap between political rhetoric and the realities facing attempts to change young people's sexual behaviour in particular contexts. Information-based approaches, the preferred option early on in the epidemic, have had little success, and great hope was held out for peer education, which is now the chosen approach in many countries. However, while peer education programmes have been successful in some contexts, they have had disappointing outcomes in others. Furthermore, their impacts frequently do not reach beyond those individuals who come into direct contact with the programme, or are not sustained over time among those living in particularly high-risk situations.

Although there is no doubt that participatory peer education holds great potential as a method for sexual health promotion among young people, much remains to be learned about how best to implement it. Small-scale peer education programmes led by members of poor grass-roots communities cannot have their optimal impacts without broader efforts to create community contexts that enable and support the performance of healthy behaviours.

In this chapter a case study is presented of a youth-led peer education programme in a Summertown school, which sought to promote condom use among young people. This case study highlights some of the key obstacles that face peer education programmes. The peer education programme used the method developed by the Project Support Group (PSG) at the University of Zimbabwe. Twenty school learners volunteered to be peer educators, and were then trained in participatory HIV-prevention methods by the Summertown Project's Outreach Co-ordinator (the same person who co-ordinated the sex worker project). Peer educators were given factual information about HIV and other sexually transmitted infections (STIs). They were also trained in participatory techniques such as role-play and the use of music to generate interaction and debate, and given an unlimited supply of free condoms to distribute. The aim of this training was to enable school peer educators to conduct informal sessions with their peers, both within the curriculum's guidance slots and in settings such as learners' lunch breaks.

The material in this chapter is framed by the conceptual framework outlined in Chapter 3. This involves a number of starting assumptions, the first of which is that the social construction of gender serves as a key obstacle to condom use. Sexual behaviour change is more likely to come about as the result of the collective renegotiation of young people's gender and sexual identities than through individual decisions to change one's behaviour. The second assumption is that a key precondition for behaviour change is the development of a critical consciousness of the impact of gender relations on sexual health. Unless people develop a critical awareness of the way in which social relations serve as obstacles to behaviour change, and a vision that things could be different, they are unlikely to be motivated to change their behaviour. Critical consciousness is a precondition for the collective renegotiation of sexual and social identities in ways that are less damaging to sexual health, as well as for the development of confidence and empowerment to be able to engage in safer sexual behaviour. Finally, such health-enhancing behaviour change is most likely to come about in communities characterized by high levels of social capital – bearing in mind that opportunities for the development of health-enhancing social capital are often limited in conditions of poverty and gender inequality.

This chapter's central theme is the way in which features of this school-based peer education programme, as well as aspects of young people's lives more generally, undermined the potential development of the critical consciousness that is so important for widespread behaviour change. These obstacles to change begin to explain the high levels of local passivity and denial in the face of a disaster of such great proportions.

## The peer education programme

The chapter first examines some of the features of the peer programme itself, before turning to look beyond the school milieu to the broader context of the programme.

### The highly regulated nature of the school environment
The aim of peer education is to encourage students to think critically about the way in which dominant social norms, as well as community and social factors, place their sexual health at risk. Among young people in

South Africa most peer education programmes take place within a school setting. Programmes depend heavily on school-based organizational structures and resources. What is the impact of the institutional environment on the functioning of the peer education programme? In the apartheid era, South African schooling was segregated according to ethnic group, with the largest proportion of teacher training and resources being directed towards white schools. Schools in the black townships were poorly resourced and frequently staffed with unqualified teachers. The standard of education provided to students was determined by ethnicity, with black students receiving poor-quality education that was believed to be adequate for their subsequent station in life as second-class citizens in the apartheid social order. There was limited opportunity for black students to progress to higher education based on the assumption that most would end up working in low-paid unskilled jobs.[1] There was also a tradition of didactic teaching and rote learning in which free discussion and argument were not encouraged among students.

Since South Africa's election of a democratic government in 1994, there have been attempts to reformulate the education curriculum in ways that move away from outdated didactic methods and to make education more socially and culturally relevant to all students. At the core of this new method is the Curriculum 2005 policy, which seeks to promote learner participation, activity-based education, flexibility, critical thinking and integration in education. However, there has been little success in the implementation of Curriculum 2005 thus far, owing to widespread confusion about the methodology among school principals and teachers, lack of teacher training to implement the approach and limited resources in many schools, all of which militate against new developments and new approaches.[2] Therefore, despite government policy, education in many township schools remains unchanged from apartheid times. Within such a context, this study's peer education programme has been conducted in a school in which pupils are subject to rigidly authoritarian school rules and didactic teaching methods, which militate against any kind of autonomy or critical thinking by pupils.

### Teacher control of the programme

The rationale of schools-based peer education is that peer educators take control of programme content and activities with support from a guidance teacher. The teacher's role is that of offering ongoing advice and support, but in a strictly non-directive way. This is part and parcel of the approach's more general goal to empower participants to take control of their own health promotion.

Contrary to the spirit of the approach, however, within this Summertown school, peer educators fell under the strict supervision and authority of the guidance teacher and the school principal. The guidance teacher retained absolute control over the activities of the peer educators and determined the times that they engaged in their educational work, also the content of their educational messages and their access to resources. Particular ways in which this was problematic for the peer educators included the teachers' insistence that they emphasized the importance of sexual abstinence in their programme, despite the reality of high levels of sexual activity among school pupils. Another bone of contention was peer educator access to the school's dedicated 'HIV activities room'. The limited access to this room, controlled by the guidance teacher, so that it would remain tidy for school visitors, was a source of ongoing frustration for the peer educators.

Towards the end of the year-long case study of this programme, some nine months after its inception, a range of teachers in the school complained that peer educators were starting to relate to adults in positions of authority in a 'disrespectful' way. In response to this, the school guidance teacher summarily disbanded the peer education team. Interviews with the peer educators and the guidance teacher highlighted very different perceptions of the reasons for this disbanding. The peer educators believed that they had been unfairly dismissed because the teacher had inexplicably taken a dislike to them. The teacher, on the other hand, reported that the peer educators had 'taken advantage' of their privileged position, and become over-confident, losing respect for the teachers and showing inadequate care for the room the school had set aside for peer education. She said that some of the peer educators had sought to enjoy the benefits of the status accorded to peer educators in the school community, while being tardy about fulfilling their HIV-prevention duties. She also reported that the school headmaster had disapproved of the fact that some of the peer educators were selected from pupils in the final year of schooling, in line with his concern that extra-curricular activities would distract them from studying for their school-leaving matriculation examination. In consultation with other teachers, the guidance teacher selected a new group of peer educators from lower grades in the school. She reported that the team now has the full support of the teachers and the headmaster of the school. At the time of writing, they had just completed their training and embarked on some peer-led activities in the school.

There has been repeated reference to the importance of peer education being conducted in such a way that participants feel they have ownership of the process. The teacher's insistence that she should be responsible for selecting peer educators runs contrary to this aspect of peer education's rationale, which would suggest that peer educators should be selected by school learners themselves. This is important not only in relation to increasing the learners' sense of ownership of the programme, but also in relation to ensuring that peer educators are people with whom learners are most likely to identify, and to whom they relate well.

*Preference for didactic methods*
Both the guidance teacher who trained the peer educators, as well as the peer educators themselves, were enmeshed within the old-fashioned

didactic approach to education which has characterized education within South African township schools.[3] Learners had no previous experience of participatory learning approaches. Pupils were given classroom access and time to do peer education during the school day. Despite being trained in participatory peer education skills (such as dramas and role-plays), the peer educators tended to drift towards the more familiar method of 'didactic' teaching. The peer educators would stand at the front of the classroom, and peers would sit quietly in rows and then put up their hands to ask questions. In instances where participatory methods such as dramas were used, they didn't form a springboard for critical discussion, as is the intention, but rather were compartmentalized to attract learner attention before didactic methods could begin. Such approaches, which see the learner as a passive 'empty vessel' to be filled with knowledge emanating from an active expert teacher, are contrary to the development of critical debate and dialogue. Such dialogue is a key process in the development of critical consciousness, as well as a precondition for the development of visions of alternative constructions of gender that are less damaging to young people's sexual health.

*Biomedical vs social content of discussions*
The content of the peer educators' lessons was framed in terms of a biomedical discourse about sexual health risks. Lessons focused on factual information about the HIV virus, how it was transmitted through the exchange of bodily fluids, and so on. Question and answer sessions after the peer educators' formal lessons tended to continue in this mould. There was no focus on the social context of sexuality, or of the way in which gender relations might serve as an obstacle to condom use.

This lack of explicit guidance on the content of peer education (explicit lessons on the way in which gender relations undermine sexual health, for example) points to one of the potential contradictions of participatory approaches to health promotion. In theory, participatory approaches seek to provide the context within which participants will generate their own indigenous critical analyses of the causes of the health threat at hand, and will reach their own self-generated solutions on the basis of such critical analyses. They are strictly non-directive, and aim to promote the empowerment of participants through the provision of the contexts for generating their own solutions to the health risk at hand, rather than through prescription for the content of such discussions.[4]

However, the ability to generate such critical analyses presupposes a very different style of thinking from that which characterizes the didactic and authoritarian style of thinking used by both guidance teacher and peer educators in this study. This could be characterized as one of the forms of 'democratic inexperience' referred to by Freire. Unless participatory approaches include explicit guidelines on the development of critical thinking, as well as explicit guidelines for the development of gender awareness, the peer education approach could simply serve to disempower young people further in two ways. First, it may simply reproduce the very gender relations that lead to poor sexual health in the first place. Second, it may inadvertently reinforce young people's lack of power in relation to their sexual health by instructing them to engage in safe sexual behaviour, without giving them any understanding of the social factors that make such behaviour change so difficult, and that they will have to resist in order to change.

This point is illustrated with an anecdote drawn from observation of a meeting of a similar peer education programme in another high school in Summertown. Small mixed groups of young men and women acted out a scenario in which a young woman, who didn't have any transport money, was offered a free lift home by a male taxi driver after an evening youth club function. Instead of taking her home he drove her to a quiet place and proposed sex. Each small group was asked to script and act out a conclusion to this vignette, which was then presented to the larger class, followed by a plenary discussion. From the researchers' viewpoint as outside observer, the common denominator in the variations of the role-plays presented by the different groups of pupils was that the older man wanted sex, and the younger woman did not, but that her power to resist was very limited. However, this 'critical' factor did not emerge in the pupils' discussions, which tended to focus instead on various strategies that the young woman might have used to deter the very insistent taxi driver, such as leaping out of the taxi and running away, or convincing him that she had AIDS and that he would get infected if he had sex with her.

In leading these discussions, the peer educators had missed an ideal opportunity for generating discussion about the way in which factors such as age, gender and lack of money had placed the young woman in this situation. However, without explicit training in critical thinking skills and in how to elicit debate around the social dimensions of HIV-transmission, such discussions are unlikely to arise spontaneously. Peer educators lacked both the critical thinking skills and the social insights to promote critical discussions of the kind that would form the basis of what Freire calls critical action.

*Gender dynamics among peer educators*
In many ways, the relationships between peer educators served as a microcosm of the same gender relations that are believed to contribute to the likelihood of unsafe sexual behaviour. Male leadership and male decision-making characterized the style of interaction in the mixed group of peer educators, with female peer educators feeling bullied if they ever challenged male colleagues. Thus, for example, one woman reported eventually resigning from the peer educator team, despite having initially been very keen to participate, because the 'guys were treating the girls so badly'.

In researchers' meetings with peer educators, discussion was almost totally dominated by two of the older male members, despite the fact that the group had initially formulated a code of conduct that emphasized that everyone should have a chance to be heard. Despite the researchers' ongoing attempts to facilitate opportunities for young women to talk, this occurred infrequently throughout the eight meetings of the group.

This situation points to one of the contradictions inherent in the peer education approach. On the one hand, the approach aims to be peer-led and to function within the context of local norms and dynamics. On the other, the approach seeks to promote the development of indigenous analyses of the roots of the problem at hand. Suggestions for addressing the problem are supposed to be generated by peer education participants, rather than being imposed from the outside. This case study illustrates the problems associated with this assumption. One cannot assume that a group of young people will necessarily have the skills or insights to engage in spontaneous critical thinking. Given the speed at which the HIV epidemic is progressing (with a doubling time of less than a year), peer education programmes need to provide far more explicit 'clues' and structured exercises to promote the development of factors such as gender awareness.

### Negative learner attitudes to the programme

As discussed, with levels of HIV infection rocketing, many South Africans have responded to the epidemic with high levels of denial and the stigmatization of people living with AIDS, or indeed of anyone with any kind of association with the epidemic. Within this context, although some learners have responded to the school peer education programme in a supportive and positive way, others have not. The latter group would taunt the peer educators, saying that their involvement in the programme suggested that they themselves must be HIV-positive. While peer educators said that this teasing was not enough to prevent them from conducting peer education activities, many admitted that they found it difficult to remain motivated in the face of such lack of support from many of their peers.

## The context of the programme

The success of HIV-prevention initiatives is most likely to be maximized when they are located within broader community and social contexts that enable and support health-enhancing behaviour change. The aspects of the school system that provide a less than ideal context for behaviour change were identified above. In this section the focus is on various aspects of learners' environments outside school that have the potential to undermine programme success.

### Opportunities for communication about sex with peers and sexual partners

Teenagers are more likely to practise safe sex if they have the opportunity to communicate openly about sex – with sexual partners, peers, and parents or other significant adults.[5] If peer education is to operate to its fullest potential, issues discussed during peer education sessions need to be exported into other areas of young people's lives and openly discussed and debated beyond the peer education context. The Summertown research on this topic suggested that school-based peer education programmes operated in a vacuum, with young people having few opportunities for the discussion of sex beyond school.

*Communication with same-sex peers*
Many young people said that they felt most comfortable discussing sex and relationships with their same-sex peers. However, for boys, such discussions tended to take the form of jokes, rather than serving as opportunities to share information about safe sexual practices. These jokey discussions served to entrench peer norms of the desirability of frequent sex. Ideally, such sex should take place at the earliest possible opportunity after meeting a potential partner, with male-centred sex focusing on male pleasure. Among groups of young women, discussions about sex were primarily concerned with the social manifestations of sexual relationships rather than the mechanics of sexual intercourse *per se*. While some young women said that they felt free and comfortable discussing sex with their friends, others reported feeling embarrassed when their female peers discussed sex, listening to the discussions but not participating in them. Young people made virtually no reference to friends of the opposite sex, so these did not constitute a source of sexual information for young people. In interviews and focus groups they referred to people of the opposite sex solely as potential sexual partners. There was also no reference to the possibility that any kind of friendship might exist between sexual partners. Friendship and sex were clearly demarcated, mutually exclusive territories.

*Communication with sexual partners*
There was generally no communication whatsoever about sex in boy–girl relationships. As discussed, despite high levels of HIV-related knowledge, levels of perceived vulnerability were low and unprotected sex was common. Research on young people's first sexual encounters found that rape or emotional pressure was not uncommon, and that foreplay was minimal or non-existent. Many young women had very negative memories of their first sexual encounter. Pressure on young men to have early and frequent sex with as many partners as possible sometimes resulted in emotional and physical pressure on young women to engage in sex. Typically young men would express a desire for sex, and young women would either go along with it straight away or else refuse for a couple of days before 'giving in'. To protect their reputations, women said that it was important not to appear available for sex (e.g. by carrying condoms). When speaking about their sexual encounters, young women generally depicted sex as something that 'just happened'. They spoke of sexual encounters as being unexpected and out of their control. Given social norms of limited discussion of sex with adults, many young women

indicated that their first sexual experience occurred before they knew anything at all about sex. In some instances, several young women said that when sexual activity began they had had little idea of what was actually happening. Within such a context the opportunities for safe sex are limited. Ironically, issues such as trust and love served to undermine condom use further. Raising the issue of condoms within a stable boy–girl relationship was seen as an indication of lack of trust of one's partner, and frequently interpreted as an insult. In short, a range of peer norms undermines the likelihood of safe sex.

*Communication with adults about sex*

Research in more affluent countries has pointed out that poor parental communication is strongly associated with poor sexual health among teenagers.[6] In Summertown, open discussion of sex between adults and young people was taboo. During feedback sessions after the research focus groups of this study, many young participants thanked the researchers for providing them with a unique opportunity to discuss sexuality with an adult 'without being punished'. Learners stipulated that while school teachers were often the exception to this rule, their sex education tended to be biological and involve the description of sexual organs, rather than dealing with feelings or relationships or emotions.

In interviews, young people repeatedly said that to discuss sex with their parents would signify 'lack of respect', and that they would never consider attempting to do this. They also said that their parents had never raised the issue of sex with them, other than mothers telling their sons to 'avoid sex, because it causes pregnancy and disease' and their daughters rather cryptically to 'stay away from boys'.

It appeared that parents tended to turn a blind eye to any evidence of teenage sexuality rather than using the opportunity for frank and informative discussion. Apart from feeling embarrassed to discuss sex with their children, parents also believe that discussion of contraception will encourage their children to become sexually active. Yet research conducted in Europe has suggested the exact opposite.[7] It is young people who have the opportunities to discuss sex in an open and relaxed way with significant adults who are most likely to postpone their sexual debut, to have protected sex, and to engage in sex in the context of longer relationships rather than casual encounters.

*Adult role models of sexual relationships*

Parents were often poor role models of sexual relationships. Many informants' fathers were absent. Fathers who lived with their families were frequently portrayed as stern and authoritarian, and also unapproachable, with little interest in the daily activities of their children and wives. Young people made frequent reference to domestic violence by fathers or boyfriends against their mothers. In short, their expectations of the quality of sexual relationships were not high.

Young people also had very traditional expectations of nuclear family relationships, so single mothers were seen as objects of pity, rather than admired for their independence and resilience. Many informants' mothers had displayed remarkable strength and resourcefulness in supporting their children and households under conditions of tremendous poverty and disruption. Young people were very positive about their mothers and the central roles they played in their lives, describing them as powerful and caring. Yet their positive experiences of single mothering did not generalize to an enhanced sense of women's agency. Despite their appreciation of their mothers' sacrifices and resourcefulness, young people did not view this as a potential new norm of behaviour for themselves. Single mothers were inevitably depicted as 'getting by' under disadvantaged circumstances.

*Community and macro-social environment*
Over the past decade there have been large-scale changes in South Africa. To what extent have these changes enhanced young people's control over their lives and increased their potential to make choices? There was mixed evidence for this. On the one hand, there were positive indications of political participation at the level of voting in national elections. Yet, in other ways, young people's living conditions did not provide the ideal context for the development of a generalized sense of empowerment and agency. They were repeatedly exposed to situations where they themselves or family members were prevented from acting on decisions or achieving their hopes. Such a context could contribute to a sense of disempowerment, which could in turn undermine young people's confidence in their ability to take control of their health.

*Poverty, lack of educational opportunities and unemployment*
Levels of social inequality in South Africa are among the highest in the world, and in Summertown, where levels of unemployment were high, young peoples' lives were characterized by extremes of poverty that shadowed almost every aspect of their existence, including their hopes and aspirations for the future. Concerns about money, food and future employment were a source of almost constant anxiety for many young people, who spoke of the stress of going to bed without food, with poverty repeatedly being cited as a source of family conflict.

In terms of educational and career advancement, young people's prospects were bleak, with a gulf between the high hopes and expectations characteristic of the 'new South Africa', on the one hand, and the grim reality of lack of financial opportunity and high levels of unemployment, on the other. Most of the young people spoken to referred to the careers they would have ideally liked to follow once they had completed their schooling, such as teaching or nursing or medicine. However, many indicated that their chosen profession would have required further education that they and their families could not afford. Many spoke of having to terminate their studies early to engage in a fruitless search for work to support themselves and younger siblings, especially those from single-parent families. In some cases family poverty had forced young people to leave school before they had completed their school-leaving matriculation examination, thereby effectively preventing further educational advancement and limiting their employment potential.

Work opportunities for young people in Summertown are exceptionally limited, even by South African standards. The economy of the town depends almost completely on the mining industry, which is responding to profit losses by retrenching staff. Very few young people managed to find work after school. A few spoke of siblings who had left Summertown and found work elsewhere. Most lacked role models for shaping their future employment, however. Most of their parents had little education and were either unemployed or employed in unskilled work. Young people had higher expectations of the job market, hoping that eventually they would find work of a more skilled nature than their parents had done, despite the lack of success they had had to date.

## Community relations

Earlier it was argued that communities high in social capital are most likely to provide contexts for the identity and empowerment processes involved in health-enhancing behaviour change. The Summertown youth study focused on three aspects of social capital: civic participation, perceived trust and helpfulness, and a positive local identity.

*Civic participation* includes factors such as voting, as well as participation in local community organizations and networks. Voting levels are said to be one important indicator of the strength and cohesiveness of a local community.[8] In this regard, the local community was a strong one. Young people were well informed about politics, and most of the informants eligible for voting had done so. Young people showed mixed reactions to the present (post-apartheid) government. They referred positively to a large-scale government housing construction programme in the area, and mentioned the construction of new schools, the tarring of roads and the provision of government pensions. These positive contributions were countered, however, by what people described as the government's poor record in creating jobs, and tackling crime – although government shortcomings were discussed sympathetically.

In terms of participation in local community groups, church membership was most common. The churches most commonly attended were mainstream Christian churches and traditional African Christian churches, although there were also some Muslims and Rastafarians among the young people interviewed. Young church members valued the church as a source of guidance ('lessons for life') as well as providing the possibility of financial assistance in times of crisis. However, although there were strong ties with the church, the high prevalence of gossip among church members precluded church as a significant source of support in times of trouble. While a few young people said they might speak to their pastor about issues that were troubling them, most preferred to discuss their problems with their families, particularly their mothers.

Many young men in the community were enthusiastic sportsmen. Owing to lack of money most of them were involved in sports such as cricket and soccer, which could be played on the streets with minimal equipment. Most were also motivated by enjoyment and their desire to remain physically fit. A smaller number of young people belonged to burial societies, political organizations and a birthday present club (a voluntary saving organization). These groups were not seen as valuable sources of emotional support, however, with young people saying that they would approach other members only with problems that directly related to their group membership, rather than more personal issues.

In relation to *trust* and *helpfulness*, levels of trust in Summertown were low. Negative gossip was a constant source of local strife between both neighbours and friends. Young people emphasized that the only people one could trust were members of one's immediate family, particularly their mothers. People were mixed in their views of the helpfulness of community members. Several suggested that families were often too burdened with their own problems and their own poverty to be of much help to anyone else. However, many did give examples of help they had received from their immediate neighbours, including the borrowing and lending of money and household goods, as well as assisting neighbours if their water or electricity was cut off when they had not been able to pay the bills. Although everyone was poor, there were frequent examples given of assisting poorer families with money, clothing and transportation to hospital. In many ways the neighbourhood often functioned as an extended family, with people watching each other's homes and greeting each other in a friendly manner.

In relation to *general community characteristics*, the local neighbourhood was seen as having three major problems. The first was the poor quality of the municipally provided services in the community. Housing was also a problem; despite the contribution made by the government housing campaign, it still had a long way to go, and many young township residents still lived in shacks rather than formal housing. The second negative attribute of the neighbourhood was crime. Young people spoke of fights, 'gangsterism' and petty theft as common features of their community. Many young women said that they seldom went out at night owing to their fear of being raped. The risks of assault were said to be particularly high over weekends and holidays when people had been drinking.

The final negative attribute of the community, already referred to above, was jealousy and gossip. Although people helped one another in emergencies, it was generally acknowledged that, in conditions of great privation, people did not want to see others making a success of their lives. Those who appeared to be improving their lot often became the focus of the hostility and jealousy of friends and neighbours.

In summary, the interviews painted a picture of a local community burdened with poverty, crime and lack of opportunity for young people. The lucky few who did manage to succeed in improving their lot often became the victims of gossip and jealousy. Levels of trust among community members were low. On the other hand, there was evidence of the existence of some local community strengths. Informants spoke of some level of solidarity among community members, who often helped each other out in time of trouble. The study community was characterized by the existence of a range of formal and informal local networks, ranging from organized churches to informal street sports groups. Furthermore, people tended to speak positively about the national government. Most informants who were eligible to vote did so, and spoke positively of government achievements. Where dissatisfaction with the government's shortcomings was voiced, this was tempered by sympathy for the difficulties of their role.

## Conclusion

What are the implications of the findings of this study for HIV-prevention among school learners? Emphasis has been placed on the importance of a multi-level approach to HIV-prevention, and arguments given that the fight against HIV in South Africa needs to involve an integration of approaches and activities over three time-scales, including the long term (as in macro-economic development), medium term (as in working to change norms of sexual behaviour through community-level approaches such as peer education) and short term (as in the aggressive detection and treatment of STIs). Efforts to promote the treatment of STIs are already in place in Summertown, so some action has already been taken at the short-term level.[9]

This research points towards the need for those concerned with HIV-prevention to give their support to a number of long-term activities, which include efforts to reduce the high levels of poverty and unemployment that undermine young people's confidence in their ability to direct their lives and take control of their health in ways consistent with their hopes and aspirations. If peer education programmes are to achieve more than superficial empowerment of their participants, there is also an urgent need for the development of channels through which participants can add their voices to a variety of local and national debates. Such debates would include those regarding which local and national education and social development policies and initiatives are most likely to provide community and social contexts that support and enable the sexual health changes peer education seeks to bring about. This would include, among other things, input into debates about poverty-reduction programmes.

However, the struggle against poverty in many parts of southern Africa has a long history, and success in this enterprise is by no means assured in the next few years. Within such a context, to advocate economic development alone as a means of addressing an epidemic that has a doubling time of about a year offers cold comfort. In the medium term, however, these research findings point to a range of interventions that could be implemented even within the context of the crippling poverty characterizing the lives of the young people in the township involved in this study. Many such interventions are already in the planning stages as the post-apartheid government battles to undo many of the negative legacies of the apartheid regime, characterized as it was by so many institutionalized measures designed to disempower young black South Africans. Many medium-term strategies are consistent with measures already being pursued by policy-makers in the educational sectors, for example. In this regard, HIV activists should throw their weight behind ongoing attempts to implement what are in principle excellent educational policies, which encourage the development of young people's autonomy and the capacity for critical thinking. The government's Curriculum 2005 strategy provides, via the 'Life Orientation Learning Area', a starting point for increasing young people's agency with regard to their sexual health. The potential impact of this 'Life Orientation' programme on young people's sexual agency is both direct and indirect. In addition to a direct focus on sexuality and relationships, the programme also seeks to improve young people's general confidence and life skills. The latter are promoted by providing young people with contexts in which they can reflect on a very wide range of life challenges, ranging from painful issues that may arise in relation to distant father figures, on the one hand, to ensuring that learners understand the links of their school subjects, marks and potential further employment, on the other.

More specifically, much work still needs to be done in developing school contexts that will enable young people to exercise real leadership of HIV-prevention programmes, and real 'ownership' of the problem of rocketing HIV levels among youth. A constituency that assumes a sense of psychological ownership of a problem is far more likely to feel empowered to take measures to address it.

Such within-school programmes could work hand in hand with social development programmes that seek to promote young people's social capital. There are high levels of awareness and interest in national politics among the young people in Summertown, and they also have sympathy and support for the ruling African National Congress (ANC) government. Within the context of such interest and respect, the ANC government's long-standing ambivalence about the causes or even the existence of HIV and/or AIDS continues to be cause for great concern. Additional causes for concern are ongoing disputes between government leaders and senior health workers and scientists about how best to deal with this problem. The South African government has been mired in bickering and disagreement about how to respond to the HIV/AIDS crisis, with President Mbeki even suggesting at various stages that the epidemic may be a fiction created by profiteering multinational pharmaceutical companies seeking to peddle toxic drugs. The failure of the government to develop a unified position – of whatever nature – about how to address the growing number of AIDS deaths, and then to exercise strong leadership in implementing this position, is worrying. More than worrying, it is particularly tragic given the high levels of sympathy and respect that young people in Summertown hold for the government.

Turning from the national to the local political scene, the research in this study has pointed to high levels of local civic participation among young people in Summertown. Within such a context, there is much scope for working towards increasing young people's opportunities to become involved in local community organizations, and in community decision-making, given the role played by 'perceived citizen power' in increasing the likelihood of health-enhancing behaviour change.[10]

Also at the local level, this research emphasizes the need for local community groups to work towards raising parental levels of awareness of the importance of open and frank communication about sex, and to start developing support for parents in this task. During the course of the research, both teachers and pupils repeatedly expressed the need for the development of a programme of evening meetings designed to support and enlighten parents in relation to the issues of youth sexuality. This is an area that is ripe for further development. Some school peer education programmes have already begun to reach out to parents, but many challenges remain, given the blinkered attitudes of so many adults to teenage sexuality. There is still a lot of work to do in supporting and educating parents so that they can play a more positive role in relation to young people's sexual health.

In relation to the peer educational programmes themselves, it is vitally important that HIV-prevention workers, peer educator trainers, peer educators and their target audiences understand the *philosophy* of peer education. This includes not only the importance of creating community contexts that enable and support the behaviour change, but also understanding of the principles underlying the need for and the development of critical consciousness. Peer education programmes need to contain very explicit and focused materials that promote discussions of the impact of gender relations on sexual health, for example. In the absence of such explicit conceptual underpinnings and materials, peer educational approaches are unlikely, however, to have any 'added value' over traditional health education, with its well-documented shortcomings.

The enterprise of promoting critical consciousness would not take place in a vacuum. As will be discussed, the post-apartheid constitution emphasizes the equality of all South Africans, specifically prohibiting any form of discrimination or disadvantage on the grounds of gender. Although currently there is a very wide chasm between ideals and their implementation, there is a legal institutional framework for the challenge of working towards the evaluation and renegotiation of gender norms that could make such a key contribution to sexual health. As is known, a significant number of township women are supporting families single-handed, both economically and emotionally. Within the constraints of very severe poverty, and against the historical backdrop of strongly patriarchal social norms, women are asserting leadership in all sorts of unrecognized ways. Although the lag between this reality and adequate recognition of the extent of women's achievements has been highlighted, this situation serves as a potential point for an increased recognition of women's ability to function independently of male control and support.

The possibility of change could also be facilitated by skilful mobilization of the young people who challenged stereotypical gender norms. Reference has been made to a small number of very religious young men who had resisted masculine norms, deciding not to have sex before marriage. There were also a few examples of young women taking control of their sexuality, through condom use and HIV-testing, with their boyfriends' co-operation. Although these counter-examples constituted a very small minority, they did exist. Some young people were self-consciously critical of the norms that governed their sexual behaviour, despite going along with them. These young people exhibited a degree of awareness of the way in which peer and gender pressures placed their health at risk. Such young people could provide valuable input into skilfully designed peer education discussions of gendered ways of being. One of the challenges for the future of peer education is to develop a peer educator selection process that identifies young people with counter-normative beliefs and values, and facilitates the articulation of their experiences for the benefit of other youth in their community.

This chapter illustrates the importance of conceptualizing school-based programmes as part of wider multi-sectoral responses to HIV-prevention. Health activists need to work hand in hand with those in education and social development departments, among others, drawing from a wide range of local and national stakeholders, including representatives of the public and private sectors, grassroots community groups, biomedical specialists and social scientists.

Against this background, what was the precise nature of the links between the particular schools-based peer education programme discussed here and the broader Summertown Project that forms the basis of this book? The existence of such links would be testimony to the Project's success in its goal of pulling together the efforts of various local community initiatives. Such co-ordination would maximize the cumulative impact of individual local initiatives (such as individual school-based peer education programmes, for example) by ensuring that activities were conducted in a synchronized way, and that strong support networks were created among groups of participants in various HIV-prevention activities throughout Summertown. In reality, however, such links were not fully utilized. At a formal level school HIV-prevention programmes were linked to the local Summertown AIDS Action Committee (SAAC), whose role was to represent local grassroots people on the Project's Stakeholder Committee. The SAAC aimed to include both learner and teacher representatives. There were, however, difficulties in maintaining consistent and continuous representation of these two groups on SAAC throughout the Project. The participation of learners, in particular, was constrained by their limited availability to attend day-time meetings through both school commitments and a lack of transport. Some links were maintained between the Summertown Project Outreach Co-ordinator and the schools. After providing initial training, this Co-ordi-nator returned to the school whenever possible to assist in monitoring school activities and planning new activities for peer education sessions. Her effectiveness in this regard was, however, limited in two ways. The first was a lack of time – the facilitation of sex worker peer education programmes left her with little time to devote to other activities. The second related to her lack of power to shape HIV-prevention policy and procedure within the schools. As already noted, the insistence of the teacher and headmaster to control the programme severely limited the extent of adolescent involvement in programme planning and implemen-tation, a situation where she was unable to exert any influence.

With the wisdom of hindsight, both the Summertown Project and the SAAC should have devoted far more time and resources to developing a systematic strategy in order to ensure that an appropriate range of local grassroots residents was consistently represented on SAAC and empowered to make use of this representation. The absence of such a strategy had at least three negative consequences. Ironically, the first was that despite its intentions to involve local people at every level of project management and decision-making, the voices of key actors in local HIV-prevention activities (including sex workers, high school students and teachers) were largely absent from the high-level stakeholder committee meetings in which key decisions were made for the umbrella Summertown Project. The second was that individual projects (such as this particular schools project) tended to operate independently of one another, losing valuable opportunities for inter-project learning and solidarity. The third was that relatively powerless social groups, such as school pupils and sex workers, were denied a vitally important opportunity to lobby more powerful groupings on the stakeholder committee about ways in which the latter's practices could be altered or improved to increase the chances of the programme's success. At the local level, the most obvious example here might have been young women lobbying provincial health departments to develop youth-friendly sexual health services where young women would not be harassed by clinic sisters. At a broader level, ideally, the Summertown Project might have served as a network for channelling young people's voices into wider regional and national debates about ways in which existing and future policies – in fields such as health and education, for example – might be implemented in ways that were more supportive of young people's sexual health. In the following chapters, attention will be given to some of the obstacles and challenges that faced the Summertown Project in seeking to pull together the variety of local HIV-prevention activ-ities, and in seeking to build links between small-scale grassroots partici-pants in small local programmes and more powerful local actors and agencies from the government, industry and civil society.

# IV

**Mobilizing Stakeholders to Prevent HIV**
Promoting Partnerships to Co-ordinate
HIV-Prevention Efforts

**Facilitating** in Project
**Stakeholder** Implementation
**Collaboration** 1

The preceding chapters have reported on two detailed case studies of participatory peer education in HIV-prevention by sex workers and young people. It has repeatedly been emphasized that such programmes are most likely to succeed with the support of parallel efforts and policies that seek to develop 'health-enabling environments' that enable and support the health-enhancing behaviour change that programmes aim for. In the interests of contributing to the development of such environments, the Summertown Project relied on a second participatory approach: multi-stakeholder project management involving partnerships across a range of local constituencies including local government, local industry, trade unions, grassroots groups, academic researchers and international funders. At an early stage of the Project it was hypothesized that two important factors would impact on Project success.[1] The first would be the strength and quality of the partnership alliances formed by project stakeholder representatives; the second would be the extent to which the Project's grassroots target audiences regarded it as relevant to their needs and interests. In relation to the second factor, the initial assumption was that grassroots community members were most likely to derive maximum benefit from sexual health interventions and services if they understood and trusted them, and identified with their goals. References to 'grassroots community members' include local township residents, mineworkers and commercial sex workers, all of whom were considered at particularly high risk of HIV/AIDS, and were thus key potential Project beneficiaries. This chapter and the next examine each of these two factors in turn.

## The nature and strength of stakeholder partnerships

*The rationale for stakeholder involvement*
The rationale for stakeholder collaboration rests on the insight that an epidemic is an extraordinary event that arises because existing attempts to promote health and treat diseases are inappropriate or inadequate. Stakeholder partnerships offer the possibility for the evolution of an

in-depth understanding of the way in which the epidemic is spreading in particular local contexts, which ideally has the potential to lead to the development of informed attempts to reshape these contexts in such ways that might limit its spread. The problem of HIV in Summertown was clearly too complex and too multi-faceted for any one stakeholder constituency to 'own' or take responsibility for it. It was through stakeholder mobilization that the Project sought to unite local people in seeking to address the problem, through the promotion of collective local 'ownership' of the problem, and by fostering collective empowerment through pooling the different skills and resources of the groups.

In reality, the stakeholder mobilization process in Summertown often reflected stakeholders' lack of understanding of the *rationale* for collective action. Stakeholders showed little interest in developing understandings of the roots of the problem in Summertown, or in pursuing the non-traditional peer education approach, or in ensuring the widespread and representative participation of local grassroots constituencies. Every stakeholder group had been involved in the discussions leading up to the formulation of the original project proposal, and each had made a commitment to participation in the collaborative process of implementing it. However, rather than working together to develop new frameworks of understanding and action, they simply continued to implement the approaches they had used before the Project, such as traditional information-based health education and sexually transmitted infection (STI) clinics, with little attempt to bring these activities into the Project's integrative framework, or to develop new forms of collaboration with new and non-traditional local partners.

Power differentials between Project employees and the stakeholder representatives meant that Project workers had little 'leverage' or 'authority' to insist that stakeholders collaborated in Project activities that fell outside the stakeholders' traditional activities or frameworks. The Summertown Project experience highlights the way in which the construction of bridging social capital is profoundly shaped and constrained by two interlinked factors: access to power and political will. Summertown stakeholders had different access to material resources (including money and the associated degree of power to exercise control over one's own and other people's lives). These differences were associated with different levels of power to exercise control over how the problem of HIV-prevention was conceptualized and managed. The Project's experience highlighted the power of particular constituencies to support selectively or undermine different conceptualizations of problems such as HIV.

# Involvement of mining houses and trade unions in the Project

As the lack of active mineworker participation in Project activities was the major disappointment facing the Project, attention is specifically focused on the nature and extent of the involvement of the two Project stakeholders that could have promoted such participation – the mining houses and the trade unions. Over the three years of the study, the mining houses showed a very patchy commitment to the three dimensions of the Summertown Project: STI control, stakeholder management and peer education. Their greatest involvement was the collaboration in the *STI control* component of the Project of both of Summertown's two mining companies. Mining industry nursing staff and doctors attended continuing medical education training courses run by the Project to ensure that their treatment of STIs was technically up to date. They gathered statistics, which contributed to attempts by the Project to monitor local STI services. Both mining houses distributed large numbers of free condoms to mineworkers, making these available from both the mine clinics and a range of easily accessible sites on the mine premises (such as hostel entrances and bars). However, while these condoms were distributed, there were few community-based efforts to ensure that miners would use them correctly and consistently.

Comparison of the surveys conducted in Summertown in 1998 and 2000 suggested that, although there was a significant increase in the number of miners who could correctly answer factual questions about HIV/AIDS, and a significant increase in *reported* condom use, these changes in knowledge and reported behaviour were not reflected in STI levels among miners. While HIV/AIDS results are not available, as stated earlier, there was a significant increase in chlamydial infection, syphilis and gonorrhoea, and in the proportion of miners who had experienced a genital sore in the past year. The only improvement from 1998 to 2000 was a fall in the proportion of miners who had experienced discharge or pain when passing urine in the past year.[2] If the Project had been successful in its goals of widespread increases in *consistent* and *actual* condom use (as opposed to simply *reported* condom use[3]), and of improvements in the uptake and quality of STI services, one might have hoped for a far more widespread reduction in STIs.

Over the three-year research period, the two mining houses varied in their degree of commitment and active participation in the *stakeholder management* process. The representatives of one of the two local mining houses played a relatively active and positive role on the Summertown Stakeholder Committee (attending 12 of the Project's 20 stakeholder meetings, often taking on tasks and actively contributing to discussions, albeit within the narrow confines of the mines' biomedical approach to HIV-prevention). This was not the case with the second mining house: its representatives attended fewer stakeholder meetings (6/20), and made little active contribution to these meetings. They seemed to interpret their role as an 'occasional watching brief' rather than active participation.[4]

In relation to *peer education*, the original project proposal stipulated that the mining houses, together with the mineworkers' trade union, would work with the Project to establish a peer education programme. This programme would systematically recruit peer educators from each shaft on each mine to ensure both optimal coverage and that all language groups were covered. This widely representative group of mine peer educators would attend a training course, convened by the Summertown Project and scheduled in consultation with the mining houses and unions. They would also attend monthly training, planning and review meetings. Mine peer educators would get time off to attend training and to conduct education activities, and would receive uniforms that they had designed themselves and modest allowances. These allowances were to be provided jointly by the mining houses and the Project. According to the project proposal, mine peer educators would work with mine management, unions and co-workers to secure industry and worker support for mine outreach activities. The progress of each peer educator, and outreach statistics, would be closely monitored in collaboration with Summertown Project staff.

A range of obstacles stood in the way of achieving the proposed goals. In the three years covered by the research, little or no peer education took place among mineworkers. Despite an awareness of the weaknesses of traditional didactic health education programmes, most mines continue to implement them as their health educational method of choice, and such approaches continue to be used in many of the Summertown mines to date. In the third year of the Project, one of the two large mining houses did employ a full-time worker to supplement these approaches with peer education at its mines. However, this worker operated independently of the Summertown Project, and as such her work fell outside the context of the holistic vision of a co-operative project governed by multi-stakeholder collaboration. Furthermore, the methods used fell short of the Project Support Group's 'gold standard' approach to peer education. Thus, for example, the few mine peer educators who were trained on the mines simply attended a peer educator training course. Thereafter they were expected to engage in their peer educational activities with no ongoing support, such as the follow-up or monitoring of peer educators, to ensure that trainees were putting their skills to good use. Peer educators were not given paid time off to conduct outreach activities. The peer education that did take place was unsystematic, often depending on the personal good will and energy of particular mine employees. There was no systematic attempt to cover particular mines, language groups and mine shafts. Furthermore, because they were not paid to conduct peer education after the training process was completed, some peer educators resented that 'the mines are expecting us to do their dirty work for free' (interview with miner who had attended a peer education training course). He said that, while he and a few colleagues had enjoyed the diversion of the week-long peer education training course, few had put their training into practice.

The mining houses' lack of collaboration over peer education has made it difficult for the Project to achieve two of its key goals in relation to peer education. The first was working to ensure that peer education would be synchronized across key Summertown constituencies (particularly among sex workers and mineworkers). The second was that all the stakeholders would work together to ensure that these programmes were conducted at the highest level of technical excellence.

The mineworkers' trade union played even less of a role in the Project than the mining houses. It made no contribution to HIV-prevention of any sort, nor did it help to drive the peer education component of the Project forward. Furthermore, its participation in the Project stakeholder management process was minimal. Union representatives attended only three (of 20) stakeholder meetings over the three-year period. While they had always been helpful when Summertown Project workers approached them for help in particular day-to-day tasks such as mobilizing miners to participate in Project research surveys, this help tended to be reactive rather than proactive. Furthermore, while they assisted with the recruitment of a few peer educators at the start of the Project, they did not initiate any peer education activities of their own, either with or without the support of the Project.

*Interviews with mineworkers*

The low level of mineworker participation in the Summertown Project, and the low level of the Project's impact on the miner workforce, was underscored in a survey conducted in 2000 at the end of the first three years of the Project. According to this survey, 2 per cent of miners reported having heard about HIV from the Summertown Project (as opposed to 66 per cent of sex workers, for example).[5] As the Project's rationale was that the Summertown Project would be an umbrella body symbolizing a unified community-wide response to HIV, this figure emphasizes the extent to which the Project failed to achieve its goals of mobilizing local people to fight HIV under one united banner.

At the same time as this survey, a series of in-depth interviews was conducted with mineworkers – which also happened to be one year after the inception of the industry-based peer education programme (conducted independently of the Project), on the mine where the industry-based programme was based. Reference has been made to the survey's finding of an increase in miners' grasp of the basic facts about HIV/AIDS (e.g. that one can protect oneself from HIV by having one faithful partner and using condoms). The in-depth interviews suggested that these basic facts continued to be embedded within the same misconceptions about health and sexuality that had been evident in the 1995 interviews (reported in Chapter 1). Miners continued to articulate a range of inaccuracies and myths about their sexual health, as well as a continued commitment to a macho notion of masculinity that undermined the likelihood of condom use. Alarmingly, the interviews suggested that five years later there were, if anything, even more misapprehensions about HIV. Several miners commented that the condoms provided by the mines could not be trusted because they were of a poor quality and had often passed their 'use by' dates. Some suggested that it was these very condoms that were causing the HIV infection. Several miners pointed to the coincidence of the spread of the HIV epidemic and the transition to black majority government in South Africa. They argued that the HIV epidemic had been engineered by whites, who were bitter about political transformation in the country and were deliberately seeking to reduce the African population by planting the HIV virus in the lubricant of the condoms.

Reference has repeatedly been made to the role of a sense of empowerment or perceived self-efficacy in increasing the likelihood of health-enhancing behaviours. People who feel that they are in control of their lives are in general more likely to take control of their health. From this perspective, a particularly worrying trend in the 2000 interviews was the mineworkers' sense of dread and hopelessness in the face of two processes. The first was the growing number of retrenchments as the mines scaled down their operations in the area, with gold becoming less profitable in the world market. The second was the replacement of many previously secure mine jobs with relatively poorly paid and insecure temporary contract work, in line with the increasing casualization of labour, and the increased tendency for the mines to 'contract out' functions previously carried out by in-house permanent employees.[6] Workers spoke bleakly about the possibility of future unemployment and the devastation that this would wreak on their own lives and the lives of their children and other dependants in a situation of high unemployment.

The 1995 interviews were conducted in the context of the general confidence and optimism that followed the 1994 election of South Africa's first black majority government. In these interviews miners were critical of and militant about their poor working conditions and right to a healthy and safe working environment. In the 2000 interviews, men were less likely to express critical views, saying that, while their jobs were dangerous, they were lucky to have them in a climate of growing insecurity, with few social safety nets. They also made reference to the increasingly global nature of business enterprises in South Africa, and the reduced ability of the trade unions, and even the government, to protect their interests. As one miner said, dismissing the possibility that the South African government might play a role in lobbying for increased health and safety on the mines: 'The government has no power in this regard. It is people overseas, people in England, who control the mines, not the South African government.'

## National and provincial government responses to HIV/AIDS

Reference has been made to the important role of 'synergy' between state and civil society in ensuring the success of local community development projects.[7] To what extent have national or provincial government leaders or actors provided a supportive context for local HIV/AIDS-related activities? At the national level, the post-apartheid constitution lays great emphasis on the rights of all South African citizens to participate fully and equally in every aspect of national and local community life, with particular emphasis on the need for women to be treated as the equals of men in every sphere. It has also highlighted the rights to health and education as two fundamental human rights. Within this broader constitutional context, the government has formulated a range of potentially very positive health and educational policies, with these latter policies emphasizing the development of young people's life skills and confidence, and placing great stress on fostering skills that will maximize the likelihood of their effective participation in social, economic and political life. Primary health care policies outline the importance of community-based health care and disease-prevention services. In short, the post-apartheid government has laid the formal constitutional and policy foundation stones for a society that would, ideally, provide a very suitable context for pursuing the types of goals inherent to the Summertown Project proposal. The challenge of implementing such policies is, however, a difficult one, particularly in the context of the deeply unequal society that has resulted from the decades of multi-layered political and economic discrimination that characterized the apartheid years. There is much work to be done in the implementation of these positive and vital policies in ways that provide a maximally supportive context for the promotion of health in South Africa.

Turning to the national government's stand on HIV/AIDS in particular, a lot has been written about repeated South African national government controversies in relation to HIV-prevention, and the absence of strong national leadership in this area. National government responses have been dogged by what have come to be referred to as the 'AIDS scandals'.[8] The first of these was the government's controversial plan in 1995 to invest R14 million (US$ 3 million) of overseas donor money in the *Sarafina II* stage musical. The musical was withdrawn after an investigation revealed confusion around administrative and tendering procedures, and after widespread public outcry at the size of the play's proposed budget, given the range of competing demands for HIV/AIDS funding. Another AIDS scandal arose in 1997 over the government's proposed involvement in the testing of Virodene (an industrial solvent hailed as a possible treatment for AIDS) on humans, despite the fact that the proposed drug had not been subjected to basic biological and animal investigations.

More recently, these AIDS scandals have been followed by various forms of presidential HIV/AIDS denial. In 2000, the South African

President Mbeki courted controversy by questioning the link between HIV and AIDS, seeking to bolster his claim with the research of an obscure and small group of 'dissident scientists' – in the face of the incredulity of most of the local and international scientific community.[9] Mbeki refused to visit the dying 12-year-old AIDS activist Nkosi Johnson, despite the child's publicized desire to meet him. In the weeks before Nkosi's death, Mbeki supporters claimed that the emaciated child was suffering from constipation, and that his foster mother had fabricated and exaggerated his condition in order to make money out of his high profile as an AIDS activist. After his death, high-profile AIDS sceptics alleged that the child had been poisoned by anti-AIDS drugs (drugs that are widely and successfully used in more affluent countries to prolong the lives of people living with AIDS). President Mbeki and government colleagues repeatedly voiced their belief that the existence of HIV/AIDS was a fiction perpetuated by international drug companies, who sought to make vast profits by peddling their toxic drugs in Africa. It was within this context that the Mpumalanga Provincial Health Department closed down the Greater Nelspruit Rape Intervention Project, which provided the AIDS drug AZT to rape survivors – on the grounds that it was breaching government policy.[10] It was also within this context that a German doctor was suspended from her job in a government hospital in Kimberley in the furore that resulted after it was found that the hospital had breached government policy by prescribing a course of anti-AIDS drugs for a nine-month-old baby girl who had been gang-raped by a group of men who believed that having sex with a virgin would cure them of HIV/AIDS.[11] This has also been the context within which, for several years, the government refused to provide the relatively inexpensive drug nevirapine to HIV-positive pregnant women, despite research evidence that this would reduce the likelihood of their babies being born HIV-positive. Leading South African scientists have estimated that about half of the 75000 infants who were born with HIV infection in South Africa in the year 2000 alone could have been saved from HIV infection had they been given proper access to appropriate drug treatment.[12] In September 2001, President Mbeki was embroiled in yet another controversy after he urged his health minister to cut the AIDS budget on the basis of a six-year-old WHO report, arguing that levels of AIDS were much lower than the biomedical profession suggested.

These are just a handful of a series of ongoing AIDS-related controversies that resulted in a lack of national government leadership in developing a unified approach to addressing HIV/AIDS in South Africa over the years of the Summertown research.[13] Already discussed is that strong and decisive national leadership may help to explain why some countries (e.g. Uganda, Senegal, Thailand and Brazil) seem to have had more success than others in addressing the epidemic. In the South African context, individual HIV-prevention programmes such as the Summertown Project have functioned out of the context of a national culture of determination to overcome the epidemic. Despite the lack of HIV/AIDS leadership from the national government, however, South Africa has a federal government system where funding for health is devolved to the country's nine provinces. Thus, even though the national government is ambivalent about the problem, some regional and local health departments have often made great efforts to contribute to HIV-prevention. This was the case in the Summertown Project, where the relevant provincial health department played an active and positive role in supporting Project activities. A department representative chaired the Summertown Stakeholder Committee for much of the three-year research period. The department also paid the salary of the Project's Community Outreach Co-ordinator who was responsible for the Project's peer education component. At various stages of the Project, it was individual provincial health department officials who had the most sophisticated understanding of the need to address HIV at the community level and not just the biomedical/behavioural levels. In other words, the provincial health department responsible for Summertown appeared to operate fairly independently of the President's scepticism about HIV/AIDS, playing an extremely positive role in the Project and often displaying greater sensitivity to the social context of health than other stakeholders.

## Degree of common vision among stakeholders

At the end of its first three years, the Project had succeeded in co-ordinating STI services in a fairly successful way across different constituencies (some GPs, some traditional healers, mine clinics, provincial clinics). Part of the success of this co-ordination exercise must be ascribed to the fact that there was already a biomedical infrastructure in place, as well as medical frameworks for understanding disease prevention. One of the reasons for the lower success in co-ordinating peer education might be that this involves replacing biomedically driven understandings of disease with more complex multi-causal models.

Stakeholders often had very different understandings of the causes of HIV, ranging from biomedical through behavioural to social explanations. Associated with these differing views of the causes of HIV-transmission was a set of diverging views about the best methods of intervening to prevent HIV. There were also varying views about whether anything could be done to limit HIV-transmission, ranging from optimism to pessimism. Stakeholders' motivations for participation in the Project also varied, some being motivated by a sense of moral outrage at the needless waste of human life and others by business interests. It was because of this lack of a common rationale that the Project generally fell back on to biomedical understandings and biomedical approaches.

## Co-ordination of the Stakeholder Committee

From the outset, the absence of a unifying vision – a result of the conflicting motivations and interests of different stakeholders – played a key role in ongoing conflicts over the co-ordination of the Project's Stakeholder Committee. The Project Co-ordinator, an internationally renowned epidemiologist, was the driving force in setting up the Project. He played the key role in the conceptualization of the Project, co-ordinating its design and funding, and pulling together prospective stakeholders. Virtually single-handedly, he co-ordinated the often fraught two-year process of consultation with the various stakeholder constituencies, which culminated in a large grant from an overseas development agency to cover the establishment of the Project and the running costs for its first three years. Once the Project was established, the overseas funding agency paid the salary of the Project Co-ordinator, who continued to be based in his Johannesburg research unit, an hour's drive away from Summertown. His tasks were to co-ordinate the employment of the Project Implementation Team, who would be based in a Summertown office; to mediate between the overseas funders, the stakeholders and the implementation team; and to co-ordinate the Project's evaluation research.

Three full-time local Project workers were employed to implement the Project from its premises in Summertown: a Project Manager; a Community Outreach Co-ordinator (to run the peer education activities); and a Clinical Outreach Co-ordinator (to run the Project's STI control activities).

The Project Co-ordinator's understanding of his role was that, in time, he would play a decreasingly central role in project co-ordination, with project co-ordination gradually becoming the joint responsibility of the Stakeholder Committee. An external consultant, who was commissioned to evaluate the performance of the stakeholder group, echoed his personal view that his co-ordination duties should gradually be shared out among the stakeholder representatives. This independent evaluator was contracted to evaluate the progress of the stakeholder co-ordination process in mid-1998 when the Project was one year old. At the time this report was commissioned, Project employees (both the Co-ordinator and the Project Manager) were battling to mobilize stakeholders into performing their roles as laid out in the Project proposal. The Project was hampered by low rates of participation in intervention activities by some stakeholders, particularly some GPs, the mining houses and the trade union.

The evaluator's report pointed to an array of structural and ideological factors that were hampering the ability of the Project Co-ordinator and the Project Manager to motivate stakeholder participation in Project activities. It pointed to the urgent need for the restructuring of the Project co-ordination process. At the level of practical management, the evaluator pointed out that it was inappropriate for one person to 'wear as many hats' and to play as many roles as the Project Co-ordinator was playing (which included Project Administrator, Trustee, Principal Research Investigator and Convener of Stakeholder Committee). To quote from the report: 'The Project Co-ordinator should not report to himself at all if possible, and certainly not as many times as he currently does. A clearer, more separate management function would be preferable for all concerned, including him.'[14]

A number of ideological differences between the Project Co-ordinator and various stakeholders were also making it difficult for him to lead the process of stakeholder co-ordination. The first related to the mining industry's sensitivity to criticism about health and safety matters. The Project Co-ordinator was a returned political exile, with a long history of participation in anti-apartheid activities. He returned to South Africa after twenty years in England following the toppling of the apartheid regime. After his return he took up the role of director of a research unit in which he was vociferously critical of the gold mining industry's health and safety record. He and researchers employed in his unit conducted research that pointed to high levels of lung disease among retired mineworkers,[15] and participated in campaigns to assist these mineworkers in getting financial compensation from the mining industry. His research unit also conducted research highlighting high levels of tuberculosis among mineworkers[16] and he criticized the industry in various public debates. As such, he was perceived by senior mine representatives as an 'enemy of the mining industry', which made it difficult to exert any influence over the mines, particularly in relation to urging them to carry out their commitments to the Summertown Project.

The second ideological difference lay in relation to the Project Co-ordinator's strong ideological commitment to a 'social change' community-mobilization approach to HIV-prevention, which was at ideological variance with biomedical STI researchers on the Project, as well as mine medical officers, who saw HIV as a biomedical problem. As stated earlier, these individuals dismissed peer education and community-mobilization approaches as 'vague social science'. Such a view, on the part of influential senior figures on the Project Stakeholder Committee did not bode well for stakeholder support of peer education, or the mobilization of grassroots participation in project decision-making.

The Project Co-ordinator had also been embroiled in a third controversy, relating to disagreements about the desirability and wisdom of accepting overseas development aid for the Project. Before the Project was set up, a senior individual in the provincial department of health had been opposed to the idea of accepting large amounts of overseas funding to build a local project. She argued that such a project would not be sustainable in the long run, and that attempts should be made to limit the amount of outside funding and implement the project with local resources. The Project Co-ordinator, on the other hand, argued that outside funding was necessary for two reasons: it would enable the Project to develop 'systems' for pulling together the complex array of constituencies involved, and it would fund the Project's heavy research component. He argued that the research component would be a 'one-off' expense, and that over a three-year period the Project could potentially make a valuable contribution to understanding of HIV through a combination of epidemiological surveys and qualitative social research. He also argued that once the 'systems' for co-ordinating the inputs of various stakeholders had been established, they would be self-sustaining, and ideally no further overseas funding would be necessary after the initial three-year externally funded period. The Project could then serve as a model for the establishment of similar projects across the country. This controversy was never resolved, and, as discussed below, the lack of appropriate health systems to co-ordinate Project actors and activities continued to be a problem throughout the three-year period under scrutiny.

In addition to these differences over issues of ideology and principle, a further range of unresolved low-level disagreements hampered the Project's progress. Chief among these was a disagreement between the Project Co-ordinator, on the one hand, and a number of key stakeholders, on the other, about the role of the media in the Project. Against the background of all these controversies, the external evaluator emphasized that the Project Co-ordinator was perceived by many stakeholders as too contentious and partisan a figure to play this central role. The evaluator also pointed to constraints facing the local Summertown Project Manager, who was unlikely to be able to wield much influence over the mining industry or the GPs for different reasons. The first of these was that, before taking up his post on the Summertown Project, he had been employed by one of the mining houses at a more junior level than the senior mine medical officers whose co-operation would be central to the Project's success. In addition, his previous job had been that as social worker, on a lower rung of the medical pecking order than many stakeholder colleagues, most of whom had biomedical training and status.

Against the background of these differences, the external evaluator's report recommended that there was an urgent need for the appointment of an 'honest broker' to mediate between stakeholders and to put pressure on those who were slow to contribute to Project activities. It was argued that this should be a person with status in the medical field, who would be able to exercise authority/persuasion over, and co-ordinate the efforts of, various local stakeholders (particularly the mining houses) and service providers (particularly the GPs). Other leading stakeholder representatives should take greater responsibility for various aspects of project finances and co-ordination, and the original Project Co-ordinator's role should be reduced to that of Principal Research Investigator, since research was his area of expertise and training.

Efforts were made to find a suitable person to take on the 'honest broker' role outlined in the evaluator's report. However, these efforts were unsuccessful owing to funding constraints. Such a figure had not been budgeted for in the original project proposal, and the Project's overseas funders were unwilling to put even more money into what was already an expensive project. As a result, the Project Co-ordinator continued to perform his many contradictory roles by default. His position became increasingly stressful and difficult to sustain for two reasons. First, the sheer pressure of demands placed on him to hold this complex and conflictual project together was too much for one person. At various stages he was working up to 70 hours a week, under conditions of great stress. These pressures were exacerbated by the fact that neither he (an epidemiologist) nor the local Project Manager (formerly a social worker) had any formal management training or skills. He also did not have the full support of many of the Project stakeholders. The task of mediating such a varied group, often with mutually exclusive needs and interests, was an impossible one. Stakeholder Committee meetings became increasingly acrimonious and often degenerated into terse or openly aggressive criticisms of decisions the Project Co-ordinator had made. People often criticized him for making unilateral decisions without adequate consultation of the stakeholders. He, on the other hand, argued that he was often forced into making such decisions because of stakeholder non-availability or apathy.

In the third year of the Project, the Project Co-ordinator managed to raise further money from an American funding agency, which was used to employ three people to assist him in work he had been doing single-handed to date: a full-time administrator, a full-time evaluation manager and a part-time senior scientist. This made his life easier and, as it became increasingly clear that the Project was a substantial, viable and important community entity, capable of attracting money, and as the problem of HIV/AIDS escalated to devastating levels locally, grassroots community members became increasingly interested in participating more actively. This development was not without controversy. What began as a fairly superficial dispute between the local community and the Project Co-ordinator's survey team, over the conduct of the Project's final evaluation survey, developed into a bitter large-scale conflict between the Project Co-ordinator and certain members of the local community. Exhausted, the Project Co-ordinator resigned and took up a research post abroad.

Despite the controversies surrounding the Project Co-ordinator, he was motivated by staggeringly high levels of commitment and enthusiasm, which did not flag over the five-year period of his involvement. He frequently became the focus or buffer for overwhelmingly high levels of anxiety, hostility and bitterness surrounding the HIV epidemic in South Africa, and for tensions that inevitably arise when such diverse groups of stakeholders, with such competing interests and viewpoints, seek to work together. Despite this, he was determined to see his commitment through, and persisted with his task. The story of the Project Co-ordinator's involvement echoes Gumede's point that the complexities and fears generated by the HIV epidemic require the intervention of people with exceptional 'passion' and staying power.

The research in this book covers the first three years of the Project. At the time of writing, an Interim Board of Management is co-ordinating negotiations among stakeholders about the long-term local sustainability of the Project. It is understood that the two local mining houses and the provincial health department will fund future project implementation, and that the American funding agency will finance a research programme centring on tests of a new method of biomedical STI control (periodic presumptive treatment or PPT) to be implemented among sex workers. Given the biomedically oriented world view of key Interim Management individuals, and the enthusiasm that has been generated around the new PPT strand of the programme, it could be possible that the Project's community focus will be diluted in favour of a more biomedical emphasis. The extent to which the Project remains committed to promoting grassroots community participation and mobilization – or else reverts to the 'top-down' biomedical and behavioural interventions and biomedical research models favoured by the mining industry before inception of the Summertown Project – remains to be seen.

## Degree of trust among stakeholders

This account of the Project co-ordination process highlights how the stakeholder collaboration process was often undermined by fluctuating levels of trust among various stakeholders, members of the Implementation Team, the Project Co-ordinator and the local grassroots community. There was also within-stakeholder variation, however. The mistrust of the Project Co-ordinator only happened in one mining house. Representatives of the second mining house took his criticism as a challenge and actively involved themselves in the stakeholder process.

The Project's relationship with the media was a deep source of contention, which generated a bitterness and friction. From the early days, the Project attracted the attention of large numbers of local and foreign media teams. The Project Co-ordinator began to develop a high media profile, which became a source of much resentment and irritation to other players. In response to this, he argued that the high profile of the Project had enabled him to raise a lot of foreign funding for Project activities and research. In addition, he pointed to the project proposal, which anticipated that the Project would become a model for HIV-prevention in other parts of the country, and emphasized that information about the Project should be widely disseminated. However, the frontline project workers comprising the local Summertown-based Project Implementation

Team objected to the Johannesburg-based Project Co-ordinator getting what they perceived as personal publicity and credit for the Project's collective efforts. Conflict also arose when on several occasions the Project Co-ordinator gave interviews to journalists without consulting other stakeholders. Furthermore, a series of irresponsible media reports jeopardized grassroots community trust in the Project. The worst damage was done by a reporter from a leading North American newspaper, who betrayed the trust placed in him by sex workers through revelation of their identities in an internationally syndicated story. This proved to be a serious setback for the Project's painstakingly slow process of winning the trust of the sex workers.

Throughout the lifetime of the Project, it was the sex workers who developed the strongest aversion to the media. Many hide their occupations from their families, so they are always particularly worried about their names or photographs appearing in the newspapers or on local television. Yet it is the sex workers who provide the opportunity for the most sensational media stories (reporters from Europe and North America appear to be particularly fascinated by sex work, and will often go to extraordinary lengths to get such stories). Furthermore, sex workers have also become increasingly irritated by the large numbers of foreign visitors (representatives of overseas funding agencies, as well as international development agencies) who have trooped through their shack settlement, with comments about starting to feel like 'monkeys in the zoo'. Thus, for example, there was great bitterness when Project workers were asked to take a senior American development agency official on a work-related visit to a sex worker peer education meeting, and this official brought her parents along. Some sex workers commented bitterly that they were starting to feel like a tourist attraction, and that it was inappropriate for an overseas colleague to have brought her parents to a work function.

A particularly regrettable breakdown in trust resulted from misunderstandings between the Project's survey evaluation team, on the one hand, and its local target grassroots community, on the other. This will be discussed in the course of the following chapter.

# 10

**Facilitating** in Project
**Stakeholder** Implementation
**Collaboration** 2

This chapter continues the discussion of the Project's attempts to pull together a very diverse group of stakeholders to work in partnership in the development of innovative and locally appropriate responses to HIV-prevention in Summertown. This discussion highlights the complexities facing those who seek to translate the powerful and convincing rhetoric of 'community mobilization' and 'multi-stakeholder partnerships' into action in the real world, where communities may often be strongly divided by power differentials, radically different world views and high levels of mistrust – all of which may become magnified in the stressful conditions presented by a major epidemic of a highly stigmatized and deadly disease.

## Degree of technical skills to run the Project

The Project's effectiveness was dramatically constrained by the over-representation of biomedical and epidemiological skills and the under-representation of other forms of technical expertise necessary to drive it forward.

### Social science and health systems development input

The first technical problem lay in a lack of expertise in social science and systems development. Although the international consultant who wrote the original project proposal was a social scientist, the Stakeholder Committee charged with implementing it was dominated by biomedically trained professionals and researchers. These people generally had little understanding of or interest in the social context of HIV-transmission or the principles of community mobilization. The committee also lacked any of the expertise on health systems development that might have facilitated the development of procedures and systems best designed to integrate stakeholders' input and expertise. As a result stakeholders often continued to work independently rather than collectively.

One way in which the Project was undermined by lack of social science input resulted from the lack of technical support for the Community

Outreach Co-ordinator. An unresolved communication breakdown led to the withdrawal of the Zimbabwean group who provided the Project with peer education expertise and support in its early stages. This was one of many breakdowns in communication that was never explored or addressed. As a result, the Project's Outreach Co-ordinator – on the basis of a short training course in peer education – had to implement peer education programmes in conditions of great complexity and danger, often with no technical support at all. She constantly expressed the need for a mentor to advise her on the dilemmas, which often arose by the hour, as she charted out new territory in the peer education field in South Africa. Although some attempt was made to link her up with a support figure in Kenya later in the Project, the nature of the support available was inappropriate to her day-to-day needs.

This situation led to friction between the Outreach Co-ordinator and social science researchers on the Project, with the former hoping that the latter might take over the anticipated mentoring role of the Zimbabwean group. The researchers insisted that they lacked the time, resources and expertise to do this, and that this was not their role anyway. Situations such as this led the Outreach Co-ordinator to express her frustration at 'useless research that is only good for publication in medical journals'.

The Outreach Co-ordinator also received no emotional support or professional counselling to sustain her in an extremely traumatic job. In particular, her task of building up and sustaining strong peer educator teams among sex workers demanded great emotional energy. Within such a context, she experienced the periodic deaths of sex worker peer educators from AIDS, as well as her role in organizing and addressing their funerals, as extremely traumatic. Although she derived limited emotional support from individual colleagues at various stages, she would have benefited greatly from greater recognition of the emotional demands of work of this nature, and from proper supportive counselling.

### Traditional healer input

A significant proportion of Summertown residents use the services of traditional healers for the diagnosis and treatment of sexually transmitted infections (STIs) and HIV/AIDS. Although the Project made an initial commitment to incorporating traditional healers into its activities, this commitment was never followed through in any systematic way. The Summertown Aids Action Committee (SAAC) included a traditional healer. Her expertise did not have special status in any aspect of the Summertown Project stakeholder management process, however. Some limited peer education was done with a small group of traditional healers during the first two years of the Project. This training was never formally evaluated or monitored, so nothing is known about its impact. In a recent series of interviews with traditional healers in Summertown, conducted as part of a separate research project, a minority of healers claimed that they could cure HIV/AIDS and were hostile to biomedical understandings.[1]

However, some traditional healers were well informed about HIV/AIDS and how to prevent it. They believed they had a positive role to play – alongside biomedical professionals – in giving patients advice about sexual health-promotion, and also in the care of people living with AIDS, including the provision of psychological support and advice about diet. With hindsight, more should have been done to incorporate healers such as these into Project activities. Their involvement might have been a useful channel through which the Project could have accessed an otherwise hard-to-reach sector of the grassroots community, for both appropriate HIV-prevention counselling and STI care.

### Management expertise

The Project also suffered from a lack of expertise in management and organizational development: neither the Project Co-ordinator nor the local Project Manager had any management training or experience. In the first year of the Project, the independent consultant evaluating the Project pointed to problems in the organization of the Stakeholder Committee. He suggested that one of the reasons for its ineffective role in driving the Project forward was that the committee's expectations were too ambitious. It was expected to provide four functions: the provision and co-ordination of professional services; the provision of support and advice to the whole Project implementation team; the mobilization of local community members in tackling HIV; and overall co-ordination and communication of all these activities within a health care system.

The consultant argued that these functions should be reallocated to smaller subcommittees, assisted by consultant specialists in various key areas. The Stakeholder Committee should meet quarterly rather than monthly. Furthermore, stakeholder representatives should not be burdened with the details of Project day-to-day management; this should have been left to the Project Implementation Team, backed up by its co-ordinating committees and professional support consultants. The report suggested that the current practice of demanding so much input from stakeholders, at a level that was too detailed and too technical, served to alienate and exclude them. As with many projects of this nature, very little was ever done in response to this project evaluation report. The problems it identified persisted throughout the three years of the Project. In short, there was no one with the training or the insight to implement the independent evaluator's suggestions. By the time the report emerged, the Project Co-ordinator was already working day and night to keep the Project going. The possibility that he might have the time or energy to restructure the stakeholder process was completely inconceivable. The local Project Manager's hands were full with Project implementation tasks. Neither the Co-ordinator nor the Manager was trained in the kind of organization-building insights that were necessary to implement the evaluator's recommendations.

*Conflict mediation skills*

Reference has been made to the breakdowns in communication, ideological and personal disagreements, structural differences and personality clashes that plagued the Project throughout its life, and severely hampered the effectiveness of the stakeholder process and Project activities. The Stakeholder Committee would have benefited greatly from professional assistance to help members reflect on areas of disagreement in a constructive and growth-oriented way. There were conflicts about the appropriate consultation of stakeholders for Project decisions, and also ongoing disagreements about who should be allowed to claim recognition for Project activities and ownership of its achievements through the media and academic papers.

Another bone of contention was the dissatisfaction of the front-line Project workers with a situation where project researchers presented Summertown Project research findings at academic conferences. The Project Implementation Team argued that it was not enough that they were cited as co-authors of such papers. It should also be their prerogative to present the researchers' findings at conferences, given that the research focused on a project that they were themselves implementing, and on the results of surveys that they themselves had assisted in carrying out. The issue of who should have 'ownership' of information about the Project was an ongoing source of often tremendously bitter conflict.

Such conflicts did not only arise between the Implementation Team and the researchers. There was also a great deal of conflict between the Project researchers themselves, which focused on issues such as the role and accountability of new research funders and new experts who joined the Project relatively late in its life. The process of analysing and writing up material from the Project's four annual surveys – which were conducted at great effort and expense, and containing valuable information about the nature of the epidemic – has been delayed dramatically. This is the result of bitter conflicts among researchers in South Africa, Europe and the USA about the content and authorship of articles and intellectual ownership of the data. At the time of writing, one group of researchers has one part of a vitally important data-set (the HIV results from the survey conducted at the end of the Project's three-year evaluation research cycle). A second group of researchers has the remainder of the data-set (including vital descriptors, without which no sense can be made of the HIV results). Because the first group is unwilling to hand over their HIV data to the second group, the Project's impact on HIV levels in Summertown is unknown two years after the survey was conducted.

In response to disagreements of this nature, individuals or groups would sometimes simply withdraw from involvement in the Project with no formal explanation, never to be seen again. At other times bad feelings would simply fester, with parties continuing to feel angry and bitter with one another over a long period, complaining about one another in private or small groups, or engaging in endless bitter email correspondences – but never openly engaging in constructive problem-solving. In the absence of formal conflict mediation skills, a great deal of time, energy and goodwill may be wasted in complex collaborative projects that lack clearly defined roles, as well as structures and systems for collaboration.

## Under-utilization of monitoring and evaluation strategies

A theme running throughout this chapter relates to the Project's lack of procedures and systems for ensuring the accountability of stakeholders to potential Project beneficiaries and other Project participants. One possible mechanism for ensuring such accountability would have been for stakeholders to agree on mutually acceptable programme goals at the inception of the Project. Donors could then play a vital role in monitoring the extent to which the Project achieved these goals, facilitating a process of annual Project monitoring, when outcomes were formally measured and, where necessary, reassessed and revised. Such a monitoring exercise could also include opportunities for Project participants to reflect on the successes and failures of the past year, and on ways in which Project strengths could be maximized and obstacles avoided in the next annual cycle. The continuation of Project funding could even possibly be linked in some way to the extent to which stakeholders made appropriate efforts to deliver on their initial commitments to Project participation.

A process of monitoring and evaluation was indeed outlined in the formal Project proposal, with clearly specified Project goals, including, for example, lowering the prevalence of STIs in Summertown by 30 per cent, and ensuring that 75 per cent of miners and other community members should receive peer education within the three-year externally funded period. The Project fell considerably short of these and other goals over this period. To follow up these particular examples, there was no significant reduction in STI prevalence among sex workers, or among the general population of men and women in Summertown (indeed, as discussed earlier, there was actually a significant increase in the preva-lence of several STIs among mineworkers over the three-year period). Only a small fraction of miners and other community members were exposed to peer education over this period. The fact that a consultant from outside South Africa had written the proposal meant that local stakeholders had a limited sense of ownership of the Project proposal. During the implementation of the Project, key Project actors and stake-holders were often unfamiliar with the proposal or with the Project goals outlined in it. In addition, the log frame structure favoured by the funding agency, detailing long- and short-term goals, and inputs and outputs, was hard to understand. As a result of all these factors, neither the Project's formal statement of goals nor the log frame played any signif-icant role in stakeholder deliberations or in shaping project activities.

The lack of stakeholder or donor interest in using these goals as land-marks for monitoring and reviewing Project progress, or improving their practice, is matched by their continued lack of interest in the Project's extremely detailed social science evaluation research component, which was very generously funded by the Project's main donor agency. These findings contain a wealth of insights about the strengths and weaknesses of the participatory HIV-prevention approaches that continue to dominate the field of international public health – in relation to both peer education and stakeholder mobilization. Between 1997 and 2000, when the research was in progress, social scientists held annual meetings with the Project's Community Outreach Co-ordinator to feed back and discuss the findings of their ongoing process evaluation of the sex worker peer education programme. However, these meetings were organized privately between the researchers and a single Project worker, rather than being part of any formally recognized Project evaluation strategy at Stakeholder Committee level. On the few occasions when social science researchers tried to present evaluation findings (either of the peer education or of the stakeholder collaboration process) at stakeholder meetings, these were tabled towards the end of long, exhausting and controversial meetings, and did not lead to any kind of useful discussion of revising project practice.

Since the end of the three-year research cycle, the Project's research findings from the social science process evaluation have been published in a number of academic journals. However, the social scientists' attempts to elicit any kind of feedback, comment or discussion of their process evaluation findings from stakeholders or donors have been unsuccessful. Colleagues who have worked in similar health-promotion or community development projects are quick to point out that projects of this nature seldom make proper use of evaluation reports, and that the Summertown experience is not unusual in this regard. This may indeed be the case. Given the urgency and devastation of the epidemic, however, and the lack of success of so many of the interventions and policies that have been devised to limit its spread, one would have hoped that stakeholders and donors might have regarded this as a special case. More particularly, one might have hoped that major players in the HIV-prevention arena – such as international donors, provincial health authorities, senior STI specialists and the gold mining industry – would have shown some interest in reflecting on why their efforts were less successful than had been anticipated in the original Project proposal. The series of papers and reports resulting from the Project's evaluation research would have been useful fodder for actors with a committed and energetic interest in seeking to understand the way in which reality intervenes between theory and practice in the HIV field. The lack of 'political will' to develop such understandings is discussed in the concluding chapter.

## Grassroots identification with the Project and its goals

A key determinant of Project success was hypothesized to be the extent to which the local grassroots community related to the Project in a spirit of ownership, identification and trust. The local grassroots community potentially consisted of three groups of black African people: approximately 70 000 mine workers residing in the mine hostels, 2 000 or so sex workers and other residents of smaller shack settlements in which sex work was conducted, and 100 000 residents of the formal township (including most of Summertown's youth). Ideally, the SAAC should have included representatives from all three groups. However, as we have seen, the involvement of mineworkers and mineworker trade unions in any aspect of the Project was minimal, and although sex workers were actively involved in implementing peer education programmes, they were never formally represented on the SAAC. As a result, the SAAC was on the whole made up of people living or working in the formal township. At the Project's inception phase, it was anticipated that the SAAC would play a central role in the stakeholder process, and that this group would provide a key channel through which grassroots voices would inform project decision-making. The SAAC failed to play such a role. A key shortcoming of the Project related to the loose constitution of the group, and its patchy involvement in the Project stakeholder process. The SAAC's interactions with other stakeholders was inconsistent, and these interactions were not infrequently characterized by confusion and bad feeling.

## Grassroots participation in the Project: What is the 'Summertown community'?

A key impetus for the establishment of the Project came from the activities of the SAAC, which revolved around a growing concern about HIV in the Summertown region in the early 1990s. This group – which lacked fund-raising skills – had made several unsuccessful applications for funding. The researchers – who had the ability to raise large sums of money, and to mobilize various sources of national and international expertise – wanted to set up an HIV-prevention project. From this viewpoint, the partnership that developed between the group and the researchers in setting up the Project was ideal: the local action group was active in the planning phases of the Project, and members of the group were employed in two of the Project's three full-time posts. However, once the Project was in place, the group's involvement dwindled considerably.

One factor that contributed to this dwindling involvement was that, for the first two years of the Project, the Stakeholder Committee (on which the local action group was to have been a significant player) met in Johannesburg, about an hour's drive away from Summertown. This was mainly because Johannesburg was the location of the Project Co-ordinator's research unit – the driving force behind the Project. The research unit had been a venue for meetings during the conception of such a project at a research level, which was some time before Summertown had been identified as a possible project site. Stakeholder meetings simply continued to be held in Johannesburg, and it was only in the third year of the Project that the meeting venue changed from Johannesburg to Summertown. Another reason for the Johannesburg location concerned the top-down nature of both the research and the health care worlds. Most of the negotiations around setting up the Project were conducted not with *local* officials of the 'stakeholding' mines, unions, research institutes and provincial health departments, but with people based at the Johannesburg and Pretoria *head offices* of all these constituencies. Again, it was only relatively late in the project that more local officials became directly involved.

As a result, rather ironic in retrospect, it was the Project Implementation Team and members of the local action group who had to set aside two hours to travel to and from meetings. Possibly partly as a result of this inconvenience, and partly because of the 'symbolic distance' implied between the Stakeholder Committee and the local grassroots group, once the Project was established these local people seldom attended stakeholder meetings during the early stages of the project.

This 'symbolic distance' might have been exacerbated by the fact that the Johannesburg-based Stakeholder Committee had little first-hand contact with the two main frontline members of the Project Implementation Team, because the three-person team was hierarchically organized, with the local Project Manager having senior status to both the Clinical and Outreach Co-ordinators. It was the latter two workers who did the bulk of the project implementation, which involved ongoing first-hand contact with local projects and actors on the ground in Summertown's informal and formal settings, whereas the Project Manager spent most of his time in the office. Particularly during the first two years of the Project, a practice developed in which the Project Manager chose to attend the Johannesburg stake-holder meetings on behalf of the Implementation Team as a whole. As a result, stakeholders had little direct contact with the experience of the Clinical and Outreach Co-ordinator implementing the Project on the ground. The potential role these two workers might have played in giving the Stakeholder Committee first-hand accounts of their work and support needs, as well as mediating between the Stakeholder Committee and the local grassroots community, was therefore limited by their lack of contact with key stakeholder representatives. None of this was helped by the lack of trust between the Project Manager and the other two workers, who believed that the Project Manager's senior status was inappropriate given the relative allocation of workload and 'on the ground' responsibility within the Implementation Team.

On occasions where the Stakeholder Committee did not support the requests or views of the Clinical and Community Co-ordinators, they often felt bitter, fearing that their manager may not have relayed their views and interests adequately to the Stakeholder Committee, or fought as hard as he could have to support their requests. Thus, for example, the Project's Outreach Co-ordinator found herself in a situation where she continually placed herself in personal danger through her work facilitating peer education in the squatter camps, and yet she had to follow instructions and decisions made by a group of rather distant stakeholder figures in an office in Johannesburg. She also felt that her work put her in closest contact with grassroots project beneficiaries, and that she was often in the best position to inform decisions concerning their interests. On more than one occasion she felt that stakeholder decisions did not reflect an adequate grasp of her working conditions, yet she had very limited first-hand contact with these decision-makers.

The third reason for the patchy involvement of SAAC, the local action group, in the Stakeholder Committee and project implementation, related to high levels of local denial, stigma and passivity in the face of the HIV/AIDS crisis. Reference has already been made to the way in which many local people responded to the epidemic with denial and stigma, constituting a virtual conspiracy of silence by many adults (parents, teachers and nurses) about the risk to young people. Some individual community leaders had done stalwart work addressing the crisis, and some local community organizations had been actively involved in HIV-prevention and AIDS care work. However, other grassroots residents had responded to the epidemic with a sense of fear, which often translated into silence and apathy, rather than a groundswell of local support for the SAAC. As a result it was less successful than it might have been in mobilizing broadly based local action and debate about tackling HIV/AIDS.

*Lack of clarity about the 'Summertown community' in Project discourse*
Reference has already been made to the Project's rather split conceptualization of what and who constituted the Summertown community. Despite the implication of the project proposal that stakeholders would meet on a level playing field, this was not the case in practice. In relation to *Project leadership*, the Summertown community consisted of the stakeholders. Because of the minimal participation of the SAAC in the Stakeholder Committee, the most influential stakeholders tended to be industry representatives, doctors, government officials and researchers. Stakeholders were invariably fairly senior members of their organizations, often with little contact or understanding of grassroots people's concerns or views. At any one time, more than half the members of the Stakeholder Committee were affluent and white, and this group very seldom included many people who had first-hand contact with the Project's target groups.

In relation to who should constitute *the target of Project activities*, a second notion of the Summertown community came into play, namely the mass of African residents in Summertown (and more particularly miners, sex workers and young people). In comparison to the members of the Stakeholder Committee, most of these were relatively poor and relatively lacking in social influence, and all were black. As conceived in the Project proposal, the mineworker component of this group should have been represented by the trade unions, but the trade unions did not take up this role in an active way. The rest of the Summertown community, including sex workers and young people, should have been represented by SAAC, the local action group, but SAAC's active membership was not always regarded as truly representative or effective, and the SAAC's participation in project activities and management was patchy.

Officially, SAAC's members were drawn from leaders or senior figures in a range of local township organizations or interest groups, ranging from teachers to religious leaders, traditional healers to youth groups. However, membership was by no means consistent over the three-year research period. There was lack of continuity in the individual organizational representatives. The size of the SAAC also waxed and waned from one year to the next. Furthermore, ironically, SAAC's membership often did not include those very individuals and groups most directly involved in the grassroots HIV-prevention activities of the Summertown Project. Thus, for example, neither the sex worker nor the school-based peer educators were ever integral to the SAAC, even though it would have been through the medium of the SAAC that they had their best chance of influencing the deliberations and decisions of the Stakeholder Committee.

To a certain extent, it was assumed that the Project Implementation Team (two of whom were local township people who had been members of the original SAAC structures that gave rise to the Project) would serve as go-betweens, linking the Project and the grassroots township community. However, this arrangement was an informal one, so the lack of clear and consistent representation of local grassroots people meant that in various conflict situations, individual stakeholders or Project workers would often bolster their arguments by claiming that they were speaking 'on behalf of the (grassroots) community', with few formal channels that other stakeholders could use to verify these claims.

It was not uncommon for local township residents to arrive at important Project meetings with no introduction, claiming to represent a key constituency (the SAAC, or a particular local organization or sometimes a more amorphous group such as 'the Summertown youth'). Such individuals would angrily and loudly express their views, and aggressively refuse to compromise on their opinions in any way. On more than one occasion, the sudden, unannounced, and frequently one-off interventions of such individuals served to derail delicate Project negotiations that might have been going on for some time, or disrupted important decision-making processes. It was tempting, on these occasions, to suspect that a so-called local representative may be an opportunistic individual in pursuit of some unspecified personal agenda. In such situations other more regular Stakeholder Committee members felt powerless to act, because no formal mechanisms had been developed for the election of local township representatives, or for ensuring putative representatives' accountability to their constituencies. Without such mechanisms, there were no procedures for other stakeholders to challenge the legitimacy of peoples' claims to represent 'the community'. Another reason why stakeholders often felt powerless to act relates to ongoing feelings of guilt about South Africa's apartheid past. In an attempt to over-compensate for years of vicious suppression of local township communities, well-meaning groups and individuals are often extremely reluctant to be seen as disrespectful of local township views. In such a situation, they prefer to remain silent rather than challenge those who claim to represent such views. This means that articulate and assertive individuals claiming to represent 'the community' or 'the youth' may sometimes be given the benefit of the doubt, even in situations where there may be doubts about their credentials.

The poor, or at best ambiguous, system of communication among various stakeholder representatives, members of the Project Implementation Team and the Project's grassroots target group led to a range of misunderstandings and miscommunications.

### Mistrust over Project funds

One particularly problematic area of mistrust relates to the large amount of donor funding involved in setting up and sustaining a project of this nature. Local people, living in conditions of severe poverty, had little notion of the expense of implementing such a project, which included the costs of running an office with three full-time workers, buying drugs for STI clinics, conducting large-scale biomedical and social surveys, and so on. When local people saw balance sheets reflecting large amounts of foreign funding, they mistrusted Project workers, with suspicions often arising that Project workers might be siphoning off some of these large amounts of money for their own personal gain. Given the tight external auditing of the funding, it was extremely unlikely that this was happening. Such unfounded suspicions were, however, very stressful for Project workers, who were already working in difficult circumstances, and highlighted the contradictions of operating multi-million rand projects in poor communities.

### Mistrust of Project researchers

Probably the most bitter of all the Project's conflicts arose in relation to misunderstandings between certain members of the local grassroots community and the Project researchers over the Project's 2000 survey. Four surveys, involving social and behavioural questionnaires, and STI testing with a random sample of 2 000 people, were conducted over the three-year project evaluation period. These surveys were to have constituted the outcome evaluation component of the Project research.

This misunderstanding involved two issues: the desire of some township residents to influence the selection of survey interviewers, and their objection to the survey team's employment of a relatively minor survey official. The bitterness of this conflict cannot be underestimated. It was linked to a growing grassroots perception that the research was not responsive to, or understanding of, the local community's needs and interests. A number of incidents fuelled this perception, including the following: the survey provided part-time employment, as well as valuable training, for 40 young people every year. Many of the young people who worked on the survey went on to find other jobs afterwards, often on the basis of the experience they had received through this work, and supported by references from the survey manager. In a context where youth unemployment was high, some community members regarded the Project survey as a resource over which they should be allowed to exercise some influence.

This desire by some grassroots community members to exert influence in the selection of survey research personnel was prompted by three factors. The first was the commonly held local perception that, in past surveys, the unpopular survey employee had given preferential treatment to his friends when he was asked to identify suitably trained township youth to attend interviews for survey jobs. The second was that certain young people who had worked on the survey in previous years had boasted to their friends that they had 'contacts in high places', which would guarantee their employment on future surveys. The research team refused to take these allegations seriously, and hotly defended their employee against these accusations. The third factor was the distinction that had developed in the popular local consciousness between two groups of young people. The first group included a cohort of young people who had worked tirelessly and selflessly to prevent HIV-transmission, and to offer care and support to people living with AIDS – for no payment. The second group included those young people who were viewed as having exploited the opportunities offered by the HIV epidemic for their own personal gain, including some who had been employed on the Project's annual surveys. Many community members were angered by their perception that these young people had been prepared to do HIV work only when they were paid for it, as opposed to their more community-minded and selfless counterparts. They acknowledged that survey workers should have high-level educational and language skills. However, they wanted to ensure that, among those who were suitably qualified, members of the first group would be given preferential access to jobs over members of the second group, as a reward for their past efforts.

Tensions over this controversy ran very high over time, with players on each side almost coming to physical blows at one stage. The survey team were driven by notions of 'independent scientific rigour' and 'technical expertise', which derived from an academic world that was very far removed from local people's everyday lives. They were adamant that they were best qualified to select survey research interviewers, and that they should be left to carry out their data collection in the way they saw best. They believed that the accusations against their unpopular colleague, with whom they had worked closely over years, often in difficult circumstances, were malicious and unfounded. Furthermore, the researchers were sceptical about the extent to which their critics were truly representative of local township views.[2]

These disagreements were fuelled by community anger about what local people perceived as the mishandling of their interests in the conduct of the previous year's survey, particularly in relation to letting people know their STI results. Owing to laboratory delays, and poor communication between the laboratory team and frontline project workers, the Project's research team had failed to meet deadlines for giving individuals back their STI results as promised.[3] On several occasions local people had to go back to the information point several times after the promised date, only to find that their STI results were not available. This situation exacerbated the stress and distress local people were already feeling about reports of high levels of sexual ill-health in the community. Such hostility was not helped by the fact that in previous years the research team had been slow to feed back overall community-level findings (e.g. HIV levels) to the constituencies (for example, church groups or street committees) who had assisted in making the surveys possible in various ways. Members of such groups had been angered to see survey results reported in the newspaper or on the television before the information had been fed back to them through local channels.

The research team was completely unprepared for the extent of the bitterness and anger that welled up against them over time. In the early stages of the Project, when there was less awareness of HIV in the community and before HIV had become such an emotive and anxiety-provoking issue in local community life, most township people had been content to let the intervention and research team proceed as they deemed appropriate. However, as local township residents became increasingly aware of HIV, and as the Project became a more visible community resource, with potential political and material influence, township people's interest in 'owning' the Project, and in exerting some degree of control over the research process, increased. The research team did not adequately understand the community's evolving attitude to the Project, or their growing desire to be consulted at every stage of the research process, and one of the reasons for this lies in local people's varying levels of apathy and commitment in relation to participation. On many occasions, grassroots township people were content to allow the Project to continue without comment. But on other occasions they were extremely keen to be involved in making Project decisions that bore the stamp of their input and influence. In retrospect, this was particularly the case in Project matters involving money or influence – not surprising in a poor community where both resources were scarce. It was also the case in conditions where local people felt that they were being treated as 'objects' of research, rather than being integrally involved in the process of data collection and dissemination. This was seen in relation to the surveys that had played such a key role in highlighting the astronomical speed at which HIV infection was accelerating in the local community.

## Conclusion

There is no doubt that multi-stakeholder partnerships provide a vital strategy for addressing HIV-prevention in less affluent settings. There has been repeated emphasis on how important it is for projects to work towards enhancing or building bridging social capital between diverse groups. Yet the process of implementing the concepts such as 'multi-sectoral partnerships', 'stakeholder mobilization', 'community participation' and 'bridging social capital' – which feature so centrally in plans to tackle HIV/AIDS in less affluent countries – is a complex and difficult one. To a certain extent some level of conflict and mistrust is probably an inevitable by-product of the ambitious task of seeking to promote collaboration among stakeholder groups that have such different views and interests. Stakeholder committees try to create relationships between groups that traditionally may not have had contact with one another precisely because their needs, interests and access to power were so very different. The multi-stakeholder collaboration process will never be an easy ride, which is one of the reasons for the repeated stress on the need for stakeholders to select representatives with the highest levels of passion and staying power.

There are many lessons to be learned, and no attempt will be made to summarize all of them here. However, a number of themes stand out. The first six themes take the form of practical lessons for those seeking to implement multi-stakeholder approaches. After outlining these six lessons, the discussion takes a more critical turn, calling for the need for a radical deconstruction of the 'stakeholder' concept. Such a deconstruction opens up the possibility of demythologizing the Project's starting assumption that such diverse stakeholders could reasonably be expected voluntarily and cheerfully to throw their energies into collaborative projects on the basis of a mutual commitment to a notion of the 'common good'. Such a demystification process is the first step in charting the key challenges facing those who seek to promote collaborative HIV-prevention programmes in highly marginalized communities: the development of systems of incentives and structures of accountability to direct and channel stakeholder efforts.

*Six lessons about stakeholding*
First, it is vitally important that stakeholders understand the philosophy of the multi-stakeholder project management approach, and the rationale underlying the potential effectiveness of stakeholder partnerships in promoting health-enhancing social change. In other words, they need to understand that, as existing approaches to the epidemic are inadequate, a new approach has to be forged, based on the principle of 'the whole is greater than the sum of the parts'. Being a stakeholder does not simply mean turning up at a meeting once a month, while the constituency you represent simply carries on doing things in much the same way as before. It involves a commitment to developing new practices and new ways of collaborating. Without such understanding a stakeholder representative's ability to contribute effectively is greatly reduced.

Second, this commitment to innovative approaches is particularly important in relation to a method such as peer education, which involves methods and understandings that depart from the biomedical and behavioural approaches which dominate the health field. If stakeholder participation is to be more than tokenism, it is crucial that the stakeholder representatives have adequate power to mobilize their constituencies to support key project activities involving novel ways of thinking and behaving. Stakeholders need either to be fairly senior people themselves or else to have the strong support of senior people in their particular organization/group, in addition to having immediate access to such senior people when quick decisions have to be made.

Third, stakeholder representatives seeking to contribute to the prevention of a problem as complex and multi-faceted as HIV need to be highly motivated individuals with exceptional leadership skills, which are defined in terms of three characteristics: they need to have the persistence and dedication necessary to address seemingly intractable problems; to be people who refuse to be intimidated by the institutional barriers, or the fossilized traditional ways of seeing things that have allowed the problem to flourish in the first place; and to be exceptionally confident and articulate in persuading their constituencies to adopt novel approaches to problems.

Fourth, stakeholder committees must have access to management skills and organizational development and systems development expertise. These are essential for the development of frameworks and methods that facilitate the collaboration of previously disparate constituencies in the development of innovative approaches. One cannot simply assume that getting a group of people around a table once a month will automatically lead to effective collaboration.

Fifth, projects need to acknowledge that biomedically oriented doctors, nurses and researchers do not automatically have the training or experience to manage complex projects. Projects of this nature depend on a wider range of skills and abilities. Stakeholder committees need to draw in a wide range of traditionally excluded groups and listen carefully to what they have to say – ranging from sex workers to frontline project employees to social scientists. Such 'bottom-up' ways of working will not always be familiar to stakeholders such as senior doctors or industrialists. It is only through the development of new ways of seeing and acting that there is any chance of addressing the HIV epidemic in a way that also contributes to the development of sustainable primary health care systems in South Africa, and improved possibilities for health in the future.

Sixth, in setting up projects of this nature, much more work needs to be done in clarifying the boundaries and constituencies of different stakeholder groups. There must be clarity around exactly which people and which interests are represented by each stakeholder group. It is also vitally important for each stakeholder group to provide very clear and transparent procedures for ensuring that appropriately representative figures are nominated to act or speak on its behalf. It is also important for particular stakeholder groups to establish transparent mechanisms whereby their representatives are seen to consult and report back to their constituencies, and to be fully accountable to the people they represent.

## Power, participation and accountability

Perhaps the lesson that stands out the most starkly of all in the Summertown experience relates to the way in which the course of the Project was shaped by power differentials between stakeholders. The 'stakeholder' concept was developed in the face of criticisms of the way in which many community development projects had historically worked with a naïve notion of communities as consisting of homogeneous residents of a common geographical space. The concept of a 'multi-stakeholder community' sought to take account of the fact that relationships between those who live or work in a particular geographical area may often be conflictual and divided in nature.

Somewhat ironically, despite its well-intentioned conceptual origins, in practice the 'stakeholder' concept is often used in a way that masks how these unequal power relations between stakeholders have the power to undermine community development goals. The same criticism can be made of the concept of 'partnerships', which features so centrally in HIV-prevention rhetoric. This was the case in the Summertown Project. There are problems in assuming that more powerful groupings will necessarily be motivated to collaborate genuinely in the development of innovative health approaches that are designed to advance the interests of marginalized groups with little social power or influence. A key flaw in the project design was the assumption that different Summertown constituencies would be equally committed to working with non-traditional partners in developing innovative approaches to sexual health promotion – or that they would have comparable capacities to do so. Again and again, the Summertown experience highlighted the way in which the deceptive neutrality of the term 'stakeholder' may serve to mask very real differences in the power that different local interest groups had to influence the course of the Project.

Thus, for example, when the rich and powerful mining industry chose to continue to privilege STI treatment and information-based health education over community-led approaches, despite having signed up to the original Project proposal, the Project had no power to influence this choice. This was also the case when it emerged over time that the mines were choosing not to meet their stated commitment to ensure that widespread and appropriate mineworker peer education was implemented within the collaborative Summertown Project framework. When trade union representatives simply failed to turn up at one stakeholder meeting after another, there were no mechanisms in place to encourage or motivate them to do so. When a biomedical scientist simply refused to hand over vital HIV data to other researchers, effectively eliminating the possibility of evaluating the Project's impact on HIV levels over a three-year period, no one seemed to have any influence over him. At the time of writing, an American funding agency (one of the two international development agencies that funded the costly surveys) continues to make some weak and ineffectual efforts to resolve this deadlock, but, in reality, overseas research and development agencies also have very limited power or motivation to influence the accountability of Project participants. These HIV survey are potentially vital data for establishing the nature of the Project's impact, and for providing information about the dynamics of the epidemic. The ongoing delay in releasing these data into the public domain arguably represents a breakdown of stakeholder accountability to the Summertown community and to those engaged in the broader HIV-prevention struggle. It also arguably reflects a breakdown of donor accountability to the British and American taxpayers, whose taxes contributed to a significant proportion of the survey costs.

Within Summertown, different interest groups had very different capacities to engage in the Project. Although, in retrospect, sex worker peer educators undoubtedly made the greatest contribution to Project implementation on the ground, in terms of the time, effort and energy they expended on Project participation for the pitifully small payment they received, their influence on the stakeholder process was minimal. While, in principle, they could have challenged this, and insisted on greater representation on the SAAC, they did not have the confidence or the capacity to do so. Located in geographically isolated settlements, with low educational levels, poor English-language skills and limited transport resources, working in a highly stigmatized profession and seeking to reduce the transmission of a highly stigmatized disease, the likelihood of them asserting themselves beyond the confines of their local HIV-prevention work was small.

Much remains to be done in conceptualizing the different types of relationships that exist within and between local stakeholder groups, with a view to deepening understanding of the way in which these relationships may often serve to hinder the goals of participatory HIV-prevention programmes. Relationships between diverse local stakeholder groups do not take place on an equal footing. Unequal power relations between different groups may impact heavily on their ability to shape or influence the process of stakeholder collaboration, and their motivation to participate in genuine collaboration with other stakeholder partners. One cannot assume that diverse stakeholders will be equally committed to supporting the Project's proposed activities. One cannot assume that powerful groupings will be motivated to collaborate in projects designed to promote the interests of marginalized constituencies with little social power or influence, or to collaborate with non-traditional partners in developing innovative approaches to health, HIV-prevention and strengthening the local community to respond to the epidemic.

Most importantly there is still a great deal of work to be done in developing systems of incentives and accountability, to ensure that project stakeholders deliver their stated commitments.[4] The Summertown experience highlights how collaborative multi-stakeholder project designs may be blunt instruments without robust mechanisms for ensuring stakeholder accountability to project goals and potential project beneficiaries. With hindsight, one of the Project's greatest weaknesses was the naïveté of its starting assumption that all parties would be equally motivated by a genuine desire to develop innovative ways of working collectively to pursue the 'common good' of HIV-prevention in Summertown.

# 'Letting Them Die'
## Power, Participation & Political Will

*Why is it that people knowingly engage in sexual behaviour that could lead to a slow and painful premature death? Why do the best-intentioned attempts to stem the tide of the HIV epidemic often have so little impact? To what extent can local community mobilization contribute to a reduction in HIV transmission?* These questions have been explored through the study of the social construction of sexuality in Summertown, and factors shaping the Summertown Project's attempts to reduce HIV-transmission. A great deal of work still needs to be done in establishing the extent to which the substantive content of the Summertown findings apply to groups of people in other countries and contexts in South Africa and sub-Saharan Africa. However, the Summertown research provides a useful illustration of the types of multi-level processes that influence the transmission of HIV/AIDS, and that may hamper the most well-meaning efforts to dislodge the epidemic's grip on so many people and communities.

In the interests of contributing to the development of a critical social psychology of sexuality, the research has illustrated the way in which sexual behaviour, and the possibility of sexual behaviour change, are determined by an interlocking series of multi-level processes, which are often not under the control of an individual person's rational conscious choice. Sexualities are constructed and reconstructed at the intersection of a kaleidoscopic array of interlocking multi-level processes, ranging from the intra-psychological to the macro-social. The Summertown interviews highlighted many such processes. Thus, for example, one's innermost needs for trust and intimacy are often symbolized by the closeness of flesh-to-flesh sex. This may become a particularly compelling option in life situations that offer scant opportunities for the development of secure and stable relationships.

Many people use the psychological defences of denial or fatalism in the face of overwhelmingly frightening threats, of the kind represented by HIV/AIDS. Such defences may be particularly common among people who are persistently faced with difficult life situations over which they have little control, or who have had few experiences of situations in which they have succeeded in meeting their hopes or achieving their aspirations. In strongly patriarchal societies, where socialization often encourages men to be macho risk-takers and to crave social power, frequent and unprotected sex with multiple partners may often be one of the few ways in which men can act out their masculinity. This might be the case particularly in situations where men, at best, work in difficult conditions over which they have little control or, at worst, have little access to jobs or money. Gender socialization may also hinder women from taking assertive control over their sexual health, in contexts where women have far less economic or psychological power than their condom-averse male counterparts. Young people, who have had little experience of ever having achieved important goals or life aspirations, may also feel disempowered to challenge stereotypical gender norms that place their sexual health at risk.

The research repeatedly pointed to the complex intersection of intrapsychic and social forces in shaping sexuality. The studies of the social construction of sexuality by mineworkers, sex workers and young people repeatedly highlighted the way in which peoples' working and living conditions may undermine the likelihood of safe sex, and why information campaigns – which target the individual as the locus of sexual health and behaviour change – have, to date, been less than effective in so many southern African contexts. In the absence of equally energetic efforts to address the wider community and social determinants of sexuality, and of health-seeking behaviour, it is not surprising that such approaches have often been such blunt instruments. The extent to which people have the ability to adopt new sexual behaviours and to safeguard their health is dramatically constrained by the degree to which social circumstances support or enable them in these challenges.

## Short-term, medium-term and long-term struggles

There is no doubt that in an ideal world one vital strategy for reducing HIV-transmission in Summertown would be to reduce the social inequalities that undermine the life chances of so many of its inhabitants. Such measures would include the empowerment of women and young people, the provision of full employment for all, an end to the migrant labour system, and health and safety legislation to protect sex workers, as well as improving the quality of education, housing and services available to those in Summertown's local townships and squatter camps. Clearly, it is vitally important that those concerned with fighting HIV/AIDS throw their weight behind efforts to bring about such social changes. However, as has been repeatedly stated, the fight against poverty and social inequalities in South Africa is a long-term struggle. A commitment to redressing social inequalities stands at the heart of national government policy in every sector, and has done so since Nelson Mandela led the first democratically elected South African government to victory in 1994. To recommend such sweeping social changes as the only way to reduce the threat of HIV/AIDS offers cold comfort to those at risk of a disease with a doubling time of a year. Against this background, it is vital that long-term measures to bring about sweeping social improvements in sexual health are accompanied by short-term measures (sexually transmitted infection or STI treatment) and medium-term measures (community-led peer education and condom distribution).

The Summertown Project was a local community initiative that sought to implement such short- and medium-term measures, through treating other STIs, educating people about sexual health risks and distributing condoms. However, rather than relying solely on health professionals to carry out the tasks of disease prevention and health education, the Project sought to mobilize the participation of a wide range of local community representatives in the achievement of Project goals. Furthermore, rather than simply aiming for *individual* health and behaviour change, the Project sought to target the whole local *community* as the locus of change – in the interests of creating local contexts that would enable and support the use of condoms and STI clinics, through the strategies of community-led peer education and multi-stakeholder partnerships.

## The gap between rhetoric and reality

Compared with many HIV-prevention projects in Africa, the Summertown Project was well resourced and on paper seemed an extremely promising initiative, containing all the elements necessary for success. Initiated by a local grassroots group, in response to a self-identified local need, it was underwritten by a large overseas development grant, and yet had realistic potential for local sustainability in the long term. Highly qualified senior scientists were on hand to co-ordinate and advise. The Project was enthusiastically launched by an appropriate and representative group of more and less powerful stakeholders, all of whom made a positive commitment to supporting project goals at its launching conferences and meetings.

Yet, even with such a promising send-off, after three years the story of the Project is a mixed bag of disappointments and achievements. The gap between the ambitious rhetoric of well-informed project proposals written by experts and the reality of life in poor local communities is often a very wide one. Many of its proposed activities and goals have yet to be implemented, consistent and widespread condom use remains low, and many Project participants feel exhausted and demoralized. The most damning proof of lack of Project success over the three-year research period is the lack of evidence for any reduction in STI levels. Many of the Project's detractors (in the competitive AIDS world, in which poorly paid local health researchers and professionals often compete bitterly for overseas funding for their work) point to the Project's lack of success as testimony to the fact that 'community projects don't work'.

One reason for the Project's lack of results to date could lie in the time that it takes for community-level projects to bear fruit. A UN AIDS review of best practices in HIV-prevention emphasizes that even the most comprehensive responses to HIV/AIDS may take four to five years to show measurable impact.[1] It may be too soon to expect results in the first three years of a community project's life. However, it is argued here that this issue was not simply one of time. A number of deeply rooted obstacles stood in the way of success. It would be premature to conclude that 'community projects don't work' on the basis of the Summertown Project, for the simple reason that many of its proposed activities were never implemented. Instead, it is argued that the Summertown Project illustrates the immense complexities of implementing community-based HIV-prevention projects in the absence of an appropriate conceptualization of the interlocking biological, psychological and social dimensions of the epidemic, the development of local skills, capacity and infrastructure to translate such a vision into action, and the development of clear and robust incentives for effective stakeholder participation.

## Political will: five dimensions

The study of the social context of HIV-transmission and prevention in Summertown has pointed to a series of multi-level obstacles and challenges facing those who seek to reduce the spread of HIV/AIDS and the suffering and devastation that it carries in its wake. Each reader will no doubt seek to draw different lessons and conclusions according to his or her particular interests and chosen levels of analysis. Below, attention is given to five of the obstacles that stood in the way of the Summertown Project achieving its goals in the three-year period of interest: variable commitment by key players; inappropriate conceptual frameworks; lack of appropriate capacity; lack of organizational infrastructure; and lack of systems for ensuring stakeholder accountability. Each of these obstacles represents a different dimension of failure of political will to bring about the social changes necessary to create health-enabling community contexts.[2] Here it is re-emphasized that 'political will' refers not only to the motivation of formal government, but also to the will of groups and individuals in the wider range of micro- and macro-social contexts within which economic and gendered power relations are produced and reproduced and (less frequently) challenged and transformed. There is no doubt that lack of consistent government leadership has been a key factor hampering HIV-prevention efforts in South Africa. However, even the most coherent and committed government response would be inadequate for tackling the HIV epidemic, and strengthening communities in ways that make them better equipped to deal with future catastrophes, without the back-up of concerted and co-ordinated responses from a range of constituencies beyond the government. These would involve not only the 'top-down' interventions of powerful groups and constituencies, but also the 'bottom-up' mobilization of local grassroots communities who have too often, to date, responded to the challenge of HIV/AIDS through various forms of denial. There has been a tendency – at all levels, from the micro-local to the international – to portray HIV/AIDS as someone else's problem, rather than taking ownership of the issue as everyone's problem. An increased sense of ownership of the problem at every level is an important precondition for the success of Summertown-type projects.

In discussing the conclusions of this book with various colleagues in the field of HIV/AIDS prevention, two different types of anxieties have been expressed. The first derived from colleagues who believed that it was vitally important to 'conclude on a positive note'. They have expressed anxiety about a conclusion that centres on the discussion of the role of what are referred to as the 'five lacks' (lack of commitment, conceptualization, capacity, infrastructure and accountability) undermining the fight against HIV. However, others argue that the time has passed for engaging in platitudes on the topic of an epidemic that is killing hundreds of thousands of people, while too many key local, national and international leaders stand by in the grip of various combinations of apathy, denial, helplessness and intellectual laziness. This determination among HIV/AIDS workers to 'put on a brave face' and 'not be too negative lest we discourage those out there doing good work' could be described as yet another form of denial that not enough is being done, and that what is being done is good enough. Furthermore, to a greater or lesser extent, there is not one of these 'five lacks' that could not, in principle, have been addressed within the design and framework of the Summertown Project. In this respect, it is argued that this book does indeed end on a positive note, in the sense that many of the problems facing the Project could, with hindsight, have been avoided. The Project has generated many valuable lessons.

The second type of anxiety was expressed by colleagues who feared that research of this nature may have the unintended consequence of being used as evidence by those seeking to argue that 'community interventions don't work'. Here it is re-emphasized that it would be inappropriate to use the Summertown Project as evidence that 'interventions don't work' for the simple reason that the intervention was not properly implemented. Furthermore, there is no longer any doubt in the HIV-prevention community that the mobilization and participation of local communities – in partnership with appropriate bodies in civil society, the public sector and the private sector – are an essential precondition for successful HIV-prevention. This point is emphasized repeatedly in various analyses of the common features of those countries that have succeeded in reducing HIV-transmission.[3] What the Summertown experience shows is that community interventions are *extremely difficult to implement* and that much careful work needs to go into setting up and implementing community programmes in a way that avoids many of the pitfalls that undermined the Summertown efforts. Many of these pitfalls could have been avoided.

The South African satirist Pieter-Dirk Uys has expressed incredulity at the levels of apathy and passivity characterizing the response to HIV/AIDS in South Africa in the slogan: 'In the old South Africa we killed people, now we are just letting them die.' At one level this criticism is unduly harsh, given the large number of well-meaning efforts that have been made by a large number of well-intentioned people in many contexts – including many of those involved in the Summertown Project. However, these well-meaning efforts and their lack of success bear testimony to the futility and the complacency of those who continue to seek to use very *ordinary* approaches and understandings to fight an epidemic that is in many ways *extraordinary*. HIV/AIDS is extraordinary in terms of the impotence of existing public health measures (STI control and health education) to contain its spread. It is also extraordinary in relation to the extent of its reach – particularly in terms of the comparative youth of the worst-affected victims, and in terms of the complexity of the social and sexual processes implicated in its transmission.

While some groups and individuals in Summertown worked tirelessly and with great commitment in furthering the Project's goals, their efforts were often hampered by lack of *commitment* by other individuals and groups. In some groups, lack of commitment to the Project's goals may have arisen from the fatalism and denial that may sometimes result from repeated individual and collective experiences of disempowerment – born out of various forms of economic and gender disadvantage over which people have little control. In more powerful constituencies this lack of commitment was prompted by a conscious decision that fighting HIV was not a high priority. This is the position that has been very explicitly taken by the President, for example, who repeatedly stated that HIV/AIDS is not as serious as many other problems and challenges facing the country. In the Summertown context, it was also taken – albeit more implicitly – by potentially influential constituencies such as the mineworkers' trade union, as well as representatives of the gold mining industry, who chose not to follow through their initial commitments to active participation in the range of Project activities.

However, even among some stakeholder representatives who were actively committed to the Project, there was an unwillingness to embrace innovative *conceptualizations* of the problem. The majority of stakeholder representatives persistently clung to biomedical understandings of disease and disease prevention, with the result that the Project was far more successful at motivating stakeholders to participate in STI control rather than in community mobilization activities. In the face of ample evidence for the role of community and social factors in shaping HIV-transmission and HIV-prevention attempts, this persistently biomedical slant supports the argument that the Project was hampered by the lack of an appropriately holistic conceptual framework. Clearly, STI treatments have a vital role to play in HIV-prevention, as do efforts to ensure that vulnerable groups have accurate information about the causes of HIV/AIDS and how to prevent it. However, there was too little acknowledgement of the need to supplement biomedical STI control and traditional health education with efforts to create community and social contexts which would enable and support increased condom use, and increased use of potentially vital STI clinics and services.

In view of the lack of commitment and appropriate conceptual frameworks to address the complex and multi-layered factors that accelerate the spread of HIV, it is not surprising that the Project lacked the human *capacity* and health systems *infrastructure* to develop and implement approaches that took account of the complex biological, psychological and social dimensions of HIV-transmission and HIV-prevention. Many would express disbelief at the claim that the Project suffered from a lack of expertise, given the range of extremely highly qualified senior scientists and doctors who were linked to the Project in various ways. However, as has been discussed repeatedly, biomedical knowledge represents only one strand of the skills and insights needed to manage a problem as multi-faceted as HIV/AIDS in Summertown. A range of other skills, in various branches of social science, organizational development, project management and conflict mediation, would have greatly enhanced the Project's impact, as would greater input by local grassroots people. There was no appreciation of the fact that the task of co-ordinating the inputs of traditionally very disparate stakeholders would require more than simply getting representatives of the different groups to sit around the same table once every six weeks for a couple of hours. There is still a great deal of work to be done in developing organizational frameworks to facilitate the collaboration of non-traditional partners. Such organizational frameworks would need to take account of the very different skills and abilities of different stakeholders, and to formulate strategies and procedures for integrating the contributions of different players, and guidelines and incentives to inform the participation of different players.

The Project's ambitious attempts to promote sexual health through the theoretically and politically sound strategies of multi-stakeholder partnerships and grassroots mobilization were dramatically undermined by differences in stakeholder power to influence the course of the Project, and by lack of trust and poor communication between stakeholder groups. With hindsight, the well-intentioned Project proposal suffered from its failure to anticipate the ways in which such differences had the potential to sabotage Project efforts. As a result, the Project was launched without adequate appreciation of the need for robust mechanisms to ensure the *accountability* of stakeholders to potential Project beneficiaries, other stakeholders and the Project donors. Furthermore, while the original proposal did indeed outline some milestones for annual monitoring and evaluation of Project activities and performance, it lacked any system of incentives to ensure that these milestones were taken seriously. Clearly, a range of unexpected obstacles might stand in the way of achieving milestones on any project. However, Project interests could be served only by the existence of mechanisms that ensured that any revisions of Project goals by any individual stakeholder were self-consciously negotiated in consultation with all the other stakeholders and the donors.

## The reproduction of social inequalities

A series of subtle social processes often combine to undermine the likelihood of successful community development and social change. According to Bourdieu,[4] many societies are structured around the unequal distribution of four interconnected forms of 'capital': economic capital, symbolic capital, cultural capital and social capital. The Summertown experience has highlighted ways in which inequalities along these dimensions influenced the community's ability to work together to ensure Project success. Such inequalities served to inhibit the development of new conceptualizations of HIV/AIDS. In the absence of these the Project made little contribution to the development of more innovative interventions, organizational systems or strategies to reduce the transmission of disease and to promote condom use.

*Economic capital* is the basic form of capital, made up of material possessions, money and property.

*Cultural capital* includes the set of social practices and skills that are slowly cultivated as a child grows up, and demonstrates his or her membership of a particular social group or class. Cultural capital includes, among other things, access to school education and higher academic qualifications. Summertown stakeholders had very different levels of access to these forms of capital. Furthermore, varying access to education and material resources impacted on people's confidence and willingness to take control of their sexual health. Such differences existed along various dimensions in Summertown. Economic capital and cultural capital were unequally distributed between industry representatives, medical personnel, Project funders and academic researchers, on the one hand, and the local grassroots community, on the other. Economic capital was also unequally distributed between different constituencies within the grassroots community, with differences between sex workers and mineworkers being the most obvious in this particular study.

*Symbolic capital* is held by individuals or groups whose voices are recognized as the most legitimate, and whose views and assertions are taken the most seriously. In this research setting, the voices of biomedical experts were taken more seriously than those of social scientists. In grassroots communities, the voices of men usually had more legitimacy than those of women, often because men had an economic as well as a psychological advantage.

Finally, *social capital* comprises the resources that derive from participation in networks of mutually supportive relationships – both within homogeneous groups and between heterogeneous groups. This research has highlighted a range of ways in which inequalities in economic, cultural and symbolic capitals shaped and constrained the likelihood that the Summertown Project would succeed in mobilizing existing sources of social capital, or in creating new sources in the interests of meeting programme goals. Far more systematic attention needs to be paid to the way in which such inequalities impact on the power, capacity and motivation of different groups to make the necessary contributions to developing effective HIV-prevention efforts. Such complexities are masked by inappropriately bland development jargon such as 'partnerships' and 'stakeholders'. Yet, as the Summertown experience shows, these differences may have a crucial impact on the outcome of project efforts.

## Whose problem is it anyway?

One of the key arguments in this book has been that HIV/AIDS is a problem best tackled through a variety of constituencies and a variety of approaches. One of the themes that has emerged repeatedly is the tendency, even among those who are most concerned about the problem, to portray HIV/AIDS as somebody else's problem. People almost overwhelmingly put the locus of change beyond their own constituencies. This failure to take personal ownership of the problem is a key dimension of the lack of political will referred to so often. At the local level, part of this lack of political will to develop effective and holistic approaches to HIV-prevention was evident in the split that developed in the Project's conceptualization of the 'Summertown community'. Frequent reference has been made to lack of clarity about exactly *who* would need to change in order to address the HIV problem. In relation to multi-stakeholder project management, the 'Summertown community' was defined in terms of high-level representatives of a range of powerful constituencies, such as the mining industry, the unions, local and national government, and a range of funders and scientists – in addition to leaders of grassroots organizations. It was this group of people who were conceptualized as the stakeholder community that would co-ordinate and manage the changes necessary for addressing the epidemic. However, there seemed to be little willingness among these powerful groups to consider the ways in which they themselves might need to change if the problem was to be addressed. Within the Project's discourse, the conceptualization of who needed to change tended to include only mineworkers, sex workers and young people (three groups who played virtually no role at all in overall

Project management or decision-making), groups who were persistently conceptualized as the objects rather than the subjects of the intervention.

In many ways, it could be argued that the acceptance of this split between powerful stakeholder managers or agents of change on the one hand, and grassroots objects or targets of change on the other (with the local Summertown Aids Action Committee [SAAC] playing an intermittent but largely ineffective overlapping role between the two constituencies) represented a profound conceptual misunderstanding that undermined the Project's hopes of success. Both groups should equally have been regarded as *both* the managers *and* the targets of change. Far more effort should have been made to ensure that grassroots people had stood side by side with more powerful stakeholders in managing the Project. By the same token, both groups should equally have been regarded as the targets of change, with as much emphasis being laid on the necessity for change by powerful stakeholder groups as by poor grassroots people. Much has been written about the tendency to locate the spread of HIV, and place the responsibility for HIV, on the 'other'.[5] This research has highlighted the way in which some mineworkers believed that HIV existed in other countries, but not in South Africa. Several young people expressed the view that HIV was the result of unusual forms of sex such as rape or prostitution, and that, by implication, they were not at risk if they had not engaged in these activities. This process of 'othering' often serves as a mechanism whereby groups distance themselves from taking any responsibility for seemingly overwhelming problems.

Among grassroots Summertown people, this denial has often gone hand in hand with the vicious stigmatization of people living with HIV/AIDS, leading many ordinary people to distance themselves from the problem wherever possible. This stigmatization has driven the disease underground in many contexts, and served as a major obstacle to HIV-prevention efforts, given that HIV-positive people are far more likely to disclose their status and seek help and advice if they live in communities that are tolerant and supportive of people carrying the virus. People living with HIV/AIDS often prefer to hide the nature of their problem out of fear – fear of rejection, but also in many contexts fear for their personal safety. People whose family members die of HIV/AIDS often prefer to tell people that they died of other causes. As a result of the taboo nature of the topic, their friends and relatives will often collude in this HIV/AIDS denial, as a gesture of support towards the affected individual or family. This distancing is but one local example of a more general tendency – at every level of South African society – to deny collective involvement in, or responsibility for, the epidemic. Such an 'othering' process was evident in, for example, more powerful stakeholders' assumptions that it was others, 'out there in the townships' or 'out there in the squatter camps', who needed to change, rather than including themselves as targets of change. They showed little interest in examining ways in which their ideas or practices might need to change in the interests of developing innovative approaches to the problem.

This 'othering' process is frequently evident in the international community's attitude to the problems of the less affluent countries in which they may conduct their business. In affluent western countries, it is increasingly common to hear of high-profile meetings where multinational companies seek to generate discussion of, for example, the way in which they can strengthen local communities (or build social capital) in their host countries – in the interests of promoting health, reducing crime or achieving a range of other laudable goals. However, when one listens to such discussions it soon becomes clear that the multinationals seldom have any intentions of conceptualizing themselves as part of their host communities. They often seem eager to fund or manage whatever change is deemed necessary among the locals 'out there', but less willing to engage in debate about how their own ideas or practices might serve to promote or undermine the strength of these communities, and impact on local people's lives and well-being in ways that have implications for ill-health, crime or whatever problem they seek to ameliorate.

In the HIV field, there is currently a great deal of concern being expressed by countries to the North at the thought of all the suffering the epidemic has caused. This has been accompanied by efforts to raise large amounts of money for the fight against HIV/AIDS. However, here again, the problem is often conceptualized as a biomedical and behavioural rather than a social one. Furthermore, it is located 'out there in Africa' rather than being framed within the context of the wider global processes that impact on health and health care in Africa, in which the international community is deeply implicated.[6] Finally, there often appears to be a worrying lack of clarity about how much of this money will be devoted to the development of human capacity and organizational infrastructure, and to community strengthening, in affected countries, rather than simply to the provision of drugs or vaccines or STI treatment programmes. The Summertown experience suggests that, in order for the impact of foreign donor money to be optimized, much thought needs to go into the development of conceptual frameworks, human capacity and health systems through which money can be channelled most effectively – in ways that lead not only to the elimination of this particular epidemic, but also to the strengthening of local communities to withstand future epidemics.

The history of the late twentieth century is replete with examples of failed but well-meaning attempts by countries in the North to 'help' countries in the South (it is not for nothing that Africa is sometimes referred to as the 'graveyard of development projects').[7] Yet the same mistakes are made again and again. Existing fund-raising efforts need to take very careful account of the complexities of feeding large sums of money into poor countries for health improvements. This point is illustrated with one recent example of an extremely important and worthwhile international fund-raising effort. At a recent G8 summit, the leaders of the world's richest countries pledged their commitment to the development of the Global Fund to Fight AIDS, Tuberculosis and Malaria. This international public–private partnership is a key project of UN Secretary General Kofi Annan, and has received pledges from a variety of developed countries and private donors. There is no doubt that this pledge represents an extremely important gesture of international goodwill, and of a genuine commitment by richer countries to contribute to the alleviation of suffering in poorer ones. Despite this, concern has recently been expressed over a number of factors. First, the pledged funds appear to involve a one-off commitment rather than the long-term annual one that would be necessary to achieve these goals. Second, the existing amounts pledged (a total of $US 2 billion had been pledged by April 2002) are said to be far too small, in the face of estimates suggesting that the achievement of these goals would require up to $US 15 billion annual assistance from wealthier countries and donors.[8] Third, the speed at which the fund has dispensed money (with less than three months between its first call for proposals and its allocation of the first $US 400 million of grants to 31 less affluent countries) has generated some concern. It remains to be seen whether or not this rapid dispersal of one-off grants in response to hastily developed grant proposals will contribute to the development of health systems, and the training of local capacity to sustain them. Finally, and not surprisingly given the speed at which applications had to be delivered, many of the applications have come from already *existing* programmes to fight HIV/AIDS, including information campaigns, voluntary counselling and testing, prevention of mother-to-child transmission, programmes to strengthen treatment, and a few requests for condoms and drugs.[9]

While each of these strategies is a potentially vitally important component of the struggle against HIV/AIDS, the speed at which proposals were written and money dispersed calls into question the extent to which fund applicants' 'country co-ordination mechanisms' will have had adequate time to think carefully about development of innovative approaches, and the types of health systems development necessary to implement and sustain these activities, or to consult widely enough with an appropriate range of 'top-down' and 'bottom-up' constituencies whose collaboration will facilitate the likelihood of programme success. One worrying possibility is that the bulk of the fund might be spent on yet more interventions that privilege old-fashioned, individual-focused, biomedical and behavioural conceptualizations of HIV/AIDS. Many of these types of interventions may indeed have succeeded in reducing levels of infection in carefully controlled academic research interventions in particular isolated contexts. However, between them, they have had little success in stemming the galloping tide of global HIV-transmission.

To paraphrase a prominent figure in the UN AIDS world: 'An appropriate response to the epidemic is not just about *best* practice, but also about *new* practice.'[10] An important measure of the success of the fund must be the extent to which it contributes to the development of successful new practices. One can only hope that history does not come to judge it as yet one more milestone in an ongoing avoidance of the challenge of developing new conceptualizations of the complex social dimensions of the epidemic, which have the potential to lead to policies and interventions that are appropriately strategic, skilful and co-ordinated.

The Summertown experience suggests that throwing large sums of money at the problem of HIV/AIDS will have less than optimal effect in the absence of the development of conceptual and organizational frameworks to enhance and sustain the benefits of this spending. Those who take the trouble to raise large sums of money to combat the effects of HIV/AIDS in Africa need to take responsibility for ensuring that this money is not frittered away on short-term, high-profile interventions that do not at the same time promote careful, logical and innovative thinking about the causes of HIV-transmission, rather than simply following the old ways of doing things. Leading public health analysts have already warned that rushing into the funding of short-term, one-off efforts could lead to long-term failures. They advocate a more modest and carefully graded series of programmes. Each country might be encouraged to start with a limited and carefully evaluated set of initial activities specifically designed to generate lessons on what capacity and systems need to be put in place in order for sustainable interventions to be implemented. These could then provide useful models for the expansion of interventions and processes across whole countries.[11] Clearly, such benefits could accrue only if current donor enthusiasm was accompanied by additional long-term commitments.

## So much more could be done: Quality and quantity

To what extent can community-level programmes ameliorate the problem of HIV, despite the fact that the problem has many of its roots in extra-community factors? A central theme that emerged repeatedly from the Summertown research was the extent to which the interlocking factors of poverty and gender inequalities served to undermine the social fabric of life in ways that facilitated the transmission of disease and undermined prevention efforts. The research also suggested that grassroots participation is by no means a 'magic bullet'. The potential for local participation to have positive health benefits depends very heavily on the extent to which local attempts by marginalized groups are supported and enabled by the efforts of more powerful constituencies, at the regional, national and international levels, and the development of health systems and organizational infrastructure to co-ordinate joint efforts. Participation has the potential to create networks of bonding social capital within marginalized communities, which is a very important component of the possibility of change. Yet such change cannot happen without the parallel efforts of more powerful groups. The Summertown experience suggests that the positive potential of such bonding social capital may be lost in the absence of the development of bridging and linking social capital. There is a need to forge links between traditionally diverse groups, with very different levels of access to material and symbolic power – but united through a common commitment to the reduction in HIV/AIDs. The extent to which the efforts of grassroots communities can result in the development of new and more health-enhancing sexual norms, and in the empowerment of people to act on these norms, is strongly influenced by the willingness of more powerful local, national and international constituencies to work with them in this task.

In principle, so much more could have been done in the Summertown context, given its well-resourced nature, and the broad range of representatives on its Stakeholder Committee. With hindsight, the likelihood of success would have been greatly enhanced by concerted efforts to generate a sense of 'ownership' and responsibility for the problem, at every level from the micro-local to the international. Much work remains to be done in mobilizing people at every level to realize that the fight against HIV/AIDS in particular, and the fight to strengthen poor communities in Africa to withstand future epidemics in general, is everyone's responsibility. It is hoped that the Summertown research has highlighted some of the ways in which HIV/AIDS is a social issue located at the interface of a range of constituencies with competing actions and interests, including international, national and local donors, experts, political leaders and business groups, in addition to grassroots communities, organizations and individuals. Locating HIV/AIDS within such a framework offers the best hope of understanding the challenges facing even the best-intentioned and technically well-informed HIV-prevention interventions and policies in the complex and multi-layered situations in which they operate. It would also lead to the development of community-strengthening approaches to HIV/AIDS that leave the survivors of this devastating epidemic better equipped to face future unpredictable epidemics, and better placed to reconstruct their life worlds once the personal and social devastation of this particular epidemic has run its course.

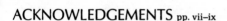

## ACKNOWLEDGEMENTS pp. vii–ix

[1] Catherine Campbell (1997) Migrancy, masculine identities and AIDS. *Social Science and Medicine*, 45(2), 273–281.

[2] Catherine Campbell (2000) Selling sex in the time of AIDS: The psycho-social context of condom use by southern African sex workers. *Social Science and Medicine*, 50, 479–494.

[3] Catherine MacPhail and Catherine Campbell (2001) 'I think condoms are good but, aai, I hate those things': Condom use among adolescents and young people in a southern African township. *Social Science and Medicine*, 52, 1613–1627.

[4] Catherine Campbell and Catherine MacPhail (2002) Peer education, gender and the development of critical consciousness: Participatory HIV prevention by South African youth. *Social Science and Medicine*, 55(2).

[5] Catherine Campbell and Yodwa Mzaidume (2001) Grassroots participation in health promotional projects: Peer education and HIV prevention by sex workers in South Africa. *American Journal of Public Health*, 91(12), 1978–1987.

[6] Catherine Campbell and Sandra Jovchelovitch (2000) Health, community and development: Towards a social psychology of participation. *Journal of Community and Applied Social Psychology*, 10, 255–270.

## INTRODUCTION pp. 1–20

[1] Summertown is a pseudonym for our area of interest. We have disguised the name of the community in order to protect the anonymity of our research informants.

[2] As will be discussed in much detail later, there are many debates about the best way to define a community. Some argue that communities consist of those who share a common identity, and others argue that communities consist of people who live and/or work in a common geographical space. In practice, for pragmatic reasons, health-promotional interventions usually target their efforts at geographically defined communities. This was the case with the Summertown Project, and it is this place-based notion of community that is used in this book.

[3] Douglas Webb (1997) *HIV and AIDS in Africa*. Cape Town: David Philip. Tony Barnett and Alan Whiteside (2002) *AIDS in the 21st century: Disease and globalization*. New York: Palgrave Macmillan.

[4] I am grateful to Roy Williams for this insight.

[5] Tony Barnett and Alan Whiteside (2001) The World Development Report 2000/01: HIV/AIDS still not properly considered! *Journal of International Development*, 13(3), 369–376. Barnett and Whiteside (2002), cited above.

[6] UN AIDS (2000) *Report on the global HIV/AIDS epidemic*. Geneva: UN AIDS. UN AIDS (2001a) *HIV prevention needs and successes: A tale of three countries*. Geneva: UN AIDS.

[7] UN AIDS (2002) *AIDS epidemic update, December 2002*. Geneva: UN AIDS.

⁸ Ibid.

⁹ Although the amount of money that has been donated to fighting HIV/AIDS by wealthier countries is minuscule compared to what is needed and what they could afford.

¹⁰ Barnett and Whiteside (2002), cited above.

¹¹ UN AIDS (2002), cited above.

¹² The relatively wealthy Western Cape province has one doctor for every 650 inhabitants, compared to the Eastern Cape where the ration is one doctor for every 30 000 inhabitants. McCoy writes of the Tshungwana clinic, serving a population of 14 000, which has no telephone, no running water or electricity and no visiting doctor. Work at night is done by candlelight, and the full range of primary health care services is often delivered with only one professional nurse on duty at any one time. David McCoy (2000) *Mail and Guardian* newspaper, 11 May.

¹³ Ibid.

¹⁴ David McCoy (2001) Keynote speaker at AIDS in Context conference, organized by the History Workshop, University of the Witwatersrand, April 2001.

¹⁵ P. Norman, C. Abraham and N. Conner (2000) *Understanding and changing health behaviour: From health beliefs to self-regulation.* Sydney: Harwood.

¹⁶ P. Salovey, A. Rothman and J. Rodin (1998) Health behaviour. In *The Handbook of Social Psychology,* Vol. II, 4th edn. (Eds) D. Gilbert, S. Fiske and G. Lindzey. Boston: McGraw-Hill.

¹⁷ C. Waldo and T. Coates (2000) Multiple levels of analysis and intervention in HIV prevention science: Exemplars and directions for new research. *AIDS,* 14 (suppl. 2), S18–S26.

¹⁸ C. Beeker, C. Guenther Gray and A. Raj (1998) Community empowerment paradigm and the primary prevention of HIV/AIDS. *Social Science and Medicine,* 46(7), 831–842.

¹⁹ P. Gillies, K. Tolley and J. Wolstenholme (1996) Is AIDS a disease of poverty? *AIDS Care,* 8(3), 351–363.

²⁰ These include the Alma Ater declaration (1978), the Ottawa Charter (1986) and the Jakarta Declaration (1997).

²¹ As early as 1998, more than half the patients of Durban's King Edward VIII hospital were estimated to be HIV-positive, for example.

²² While little has been written about the demands of home-based care for AIDS patients in South Africa, research in countries such as Tanzania, where the epidemic is in its more advanced stages, paints a grim picture of the challenges of nursing a dying AIDS patient. Soori Nnko, Betty Chiduo, Flora Wilson, Wences Msuya and Gabriel Mwaluko (2000) Tanzania: AIDS care – learning from experience. *Review of African Political Economy,* 86, 547–557.

²³ Jonathan Crush and Wilmott James (Eds) (1995) *Crossing boundaries: Mine migrancy in a democratic South Africa.* Cape Town: IDRC/IDASA.

²⁴ Jonathan Crush, Theresa Ulicki, Teke Tseane and Elizabeth Jansen van Vuuren (2001) Undermining labour: The rise of sub-contracting in South African gold mines. *Journal of Southern African Studies,* 27(1), 5–31.

²⁵ Brian Williams, Denise Gilgen, Catherine Campbell, Dirk Taljaard and Catherine MacPhail (2000) *The natural history of HIV/AIDS in South Africa: A biomedical and social survey.* Johannesburg: CSIR. At the time this survey was conducted, the exchange rate of South African rands to British pounds was R10 to £1.

²⁶ Louisiana Lush (2000) Integrating HIV/STI and primary health care services: International policy developments and national responses with special reference to South Africa. Unpublished PhD thesis, London School of Hygiene and Tropical Medicine.

²⁷ Dennis J. Dobbs (2000) *Summertown: South Africa. Results of the Second Community-based Survey.* Report to US Population Council, New York.

²⁸ See, for example: Helen Schneider and Joanne Stein (2000) Implementing AIDS policy in post-apartheid South Africa. *Social Science and Medicine,* 52, 723–731.

²⁹ I am grateful to Brian Williams for this point.

³⁰ Brian Williams and Eleanor Gouws (2001) The epidemiology of AIDS in South Africa. *Philosophical Transactions of the Royal Society.* B, 356: 1077–1086.

# CHAPTER 1 pp. 23–35

[1] This research was conducted by the author and a colleague, Prof. Brian Williams, who was director of the Johannesburg-based Epidemiology Research Institute, a research unit charged with conducting research into the health and safety of mineworkers.

[2] J. Decosas (1994) The answer to AIDS lies in united commitment. *AIDS Analysis Africa (Southern African Edition)*, 5(1), 3–4.

[3] Lettie La Grange (1996) HIV infected individuals in industries at a high risk for TB: A rejoinder to London, Maartens, Myers and Bereleowitz. *Occupational Health South Africa*, 2, 8–10.

[4] Anthony Zwi, Sharon Fonn and Malcolm Steinberg (1988) Occupational health and safety in South Africa: The perspectives of capital, state and the unions. *Social Science and Medicine*, 27(7), 691–702.

[5] Although about 22% of miners were estimated to be HIV-positive at the time of our interviews, at the early stage of the epidemic, first-hand contact with cases of full-blown AIDS was very limited.

[6] Jean Comaroff (1980) Healing and the cultural order: The case of the Barolong Boo Ratshidi of Southern Africa. *American Ethnologist*, 7, 637–657.

[7] The Hon. R. Leon, A. Davies, M. Salamon and J. Davies (1995) *Commission of inquiry into safety and health in the mining industry*. Department of Mineral and Energy Affairs, Pretoria. M. Molapo (1995) Job stress, health and perceptions of migrant mineworkers. In Jonathan Crush and Wilmott James (Eds) *Crossing boundaries: Mine migrancy in a democratic South Africa*. Cape Town: IDRC/IDASA, pp. 88–100.

[8] An underground worker has a 2.9% chance of being killed in a work-related accident and a 42% chance of suffering a reportable injury in a 20-year working life. This figure was calculated from the average fatality and reportable injury rates published by the South African Chamber of Mines for the 10-year period 1984–93. Chamber of Mines (1993) *Statistical Tables 1993*. Chamber of Mines, Johannesburg.

[9] Albert Bandura (1996) *Self-efficacy in changing societies*. Cambridge: Cambridge University Press.

[10] The incidence of tuberculosis on South African mines increased from 620 per 100 000 workers per year in 1988 to 1 070 per 100 000 workers per year in 1992. R. Packard and D. Coetzee (1995) White plague: black labour revisited: TB and the mining industry. In Jonathan Crush and Wilmott James (Eds) *Crossing boundaries: Mine migrancy in a democratic South Africa*. Cape Town: IDRC/IDASA, pp. 101–115.

[11] Dunbar Moodie (1994) has written in detail about the role of masculinity in shaping South African mineworkers' general social identities. He comments that an aggressive and macho masculinity forms a pillar of identity formation among large collectivities of working men in a range of contexts and continents, and is certainly not peculiar to southern Africa, or to mineworkers. T. Dunbar Moodie (1994) *Going for gold: Men, mines and migration*. Johannesburg: Witwatersrand University Press.

[12] Ibid. Ari Sitas (1985) From grassroots control to democracy: A case study of the impact of trade unionism on migrant workers' cultural formations. *Social Dynamics*, 11(1), 32–43.

[13] While same-sex relationships in the form of formal 'mine marriages' were a common feature of life in the mine hostels until the 1970s (Moodie 1994), miners said these were now less common. In interviews, female sex workers referred to a recent trend where young men were starting to sell sex to miners in the veld in competition with women. They said that this form of sex tended to be inter-crural in nature (with men rubbing their penises between the young men's thighs) rather than involving any form of bodily penetration. As such, sex workers said that some more health-conscious mineworkers regarded this as a safer sex strategy. This practice was not mentioned by mineworkers.

[14] A. Prieur (1990) Norwegian gay men: Reasons for the continued practice of unsafe sex. *AIDS Education and Prevention*, 2(2), 109–115.

[15] D. Mechanic (1990) Promoting health. *Society*, 16–22 January.

[16] Moodie (1994), cited above.

[17] Campbell (1992) discusses the range of ways in which men might seek to compensate for the loss of masculinity as more traditional patriarchal family structures (in which men had a great deal of power over women and children) are eroded. Catherine Campbell (1992) Learning to kill? The family, masculinity and political violence in Natal. *Journal of Southern African Studies*, 18(3), 614–628.

[18] M. Hayes (1992) On the epistemology of risk: Language, logic and social science. *Social Science and Medicine*, 35(4), 401–407.

[19] Kim M. Blankenship, Sarah J. Bray and Michael H. Merson (2000) Structural interventions in public health. *AIDS*, 14 (suppl. 1), S11–S21. Richard Parker, Delia Easton and Charles H. Klein (2000) Structural barriers and facilitators in HIV prevention: A review of international research. *AIDS*, 14 (suppl. 1), S22–S32.

[20] Oussama Tawil, Annette Verster and Kevin O'Reilly (1995) Enabling approaches for HIV/AIDS promotion: Can we modify the environment and minimise the risk? *AIDS*, 9, 1299–1306.

## CHAPTER 2 pp. 36–44

[1] Including the author of this book, and under the leadership of Brian Williams.

[2] Catherine Campbell and Brian Williams (1999) Beyond the biomedical and behavioural: Towards an integrated approach to HIV-prevention in the southern African mining industry. *Social Science and Medicine*, 48, 1625–1639.

[3] Anthony Zwi and Deborah Bachmayer (1990) HIV and Aids in South Africa: What is an appropriate public health response? *Health Policy and Planning*, 5, 316–326.

[4] UN AIDS (2001b) *Innovative approaches to HIV prevention: Selected case studies*. Geneva: UN AIDS. UN AIDS (2001a) *HIV prevention needs and successes: A tale of three countries*. Geneva: UN AIDS.

[5] Claudio Lanata (2001) Children's health in developing countries: Issues of coping, child neglect and marginalization. In David Leon and Gill Walt (Eds) *Poverty, inequality and health: An international perspective*. Oxford: Oxford University Press.

[6] For a detailed discussion of different health promotional approaches, see Chapter 15 of David Marks, Michael Murray, Brian Evans and Carla Willig (1999) *Health psychology: Theory and practice*. London: Sage.

[7] UN AIDS (1999) *Peer education and HIV/AIDS: Concepts, uses and challenges*. Geneva: UN AIDS. N. Janz (1996) Evaluation of 37 AIDS Prevention Projects: Successful approaches and barriers to program effectiveness. *Health Education Quarterly*, 23, 80–97.

[8] David Wilson (1995) Community peer education to prevent STD/HIV/AIDS among women in Zimbabwe and Zambia. Unpublished report by the Project Support Group, Psychology Department, University of Zimbabwe.

[9] Nolene Dube and David Wilson (1999) Peer education programmes. In Brian Williams, Catherine Campbell and Catherine MacPhail (Eds) *Managing HIV/AIDS in South Africa: Lessons from industrial settings*. Johannesburg: CSIR. N. Ngugi, D. Wilson, J. Sebstad, F. Plummer and S. Moses (1996) Focused peer-mediated educational programmes among female sex workers to reduce sexually transmitted disease and human immunodeficiency virus transmission in Kenya and Zimbabwe. *Journal of Infectious Diseases*, 174 (suppl. 2), S240–S247.

[10] Ideally, an outcome evaluation would also compare the intervention site with a site that had not been exposed to the intervention. In Summertown, such a research design was not possible, either on ethical or logistical grounds.

[11] P. Aggleton, A. Young, D. Moody, M. Kapila and M. Pye (1992) *Does it work? Perspectives on the evaluation of HIV/AIDS health promotion*. London: Health Education Authority.

[12] Brian Williams, Dirk Taljaard, Catherine Campbell and others (forthcoming) Changing patterns of knowledge, reported behaviour and sexually transmitted infections in a South African mining community. *AIDS*.

# CHAPTER 3 pp. 45–60

[1] As already stated, this chapter is likely to be of the greatest interest to academic readers. Non-academic readers may want to take the option of leaving this chapter out, and proceeding directly to Chapter 4.

[2] C. Beeker, C. Guenther Gray and A. Raj (1998) Community empowerment paradigm and the primary prevention of HIV/AIDS. *Social Science and Medicine*, 46(7), 831–842.

[3] UN AIDS (1999) *Peer education and HIV/AIDS: Concepts, uses and challenges*. Geneva: UN AIDS.

[4] G. Turner and J. Shepherd (1999) A method in search of a theory: Peer education and health promotion. *Health Education Research*, 14(2), 235–247.

[5] Kathryn Milburn (1995) A critical review of peer education with young people with special reference to sexual health. *Health Education Research: Theory and Practice*, 10(4), 407–420.

[6] Catherine MacPhail and Catherine Campbell (1999) Evaluating HIV-prevention programmes: Do current indicators do justice to advances in intervention? *South African Journal of Psychology*, 29(4), 149–165.

[7] Jan Stockdale (1995) The self and media messages: Match or mismatch? In Ivana Marková and Rob Farr (Eds) *Representations of health, illness and handicap*. London: Harwood, pp. 31–48.

[8] Michael Billig (1996) *Arguing and thinking*. Cambridge: Cambridge University Press.

[9] Janet Holland (1998) *The male in the head*. London: Tufnell Press.

[10] Stuart Hall (1992) Cultural identity in question. In S. Hall, D. Held and T. McGrew, *Modernity and its futures*. Cambridge: Polity Press, pp. 273–316.

[11] Nina Wallerstein (1992) Powerlessness, empowerment and health: Implications for health promotion programmes. *American Journal of Health Promotion*, 6(3), 197–205.

[12] Paulo Freire (1970/1993a) *The pedagogy of the oppressed*. London: Penguin. Paulo Freire (1973/1993b) *Education for critical consciousness*. New York: Continuum.

[13] Freire (1993b), p. 19.

[14] Ibid., p. 23.

[15] Fran Baum (1999a) Editorial. Social capital: Is it good for your health? Issues for a public health agenda. *Journal of Epidemiology and Community Health*, 53(4), 195–196.

[16] Catherine Campbell (2000) Social capital and health: Contextualising health promotion within local community networks. In Steve Baron, John Field, and Tom Schuller (Eds) *Social capital: Critical perspectives*. Oxford: Oxford University Press, pp. 182–196. Catherine Campbell, Rachel Wood and Moira Kelly (1999) *Social capital and health*. London: Health Education Authority.

[17] Mildred Blaxter (2000) Medical sociology at the start of the new millennium. *Social Science and Medicine*, 51, 1139–1142.

[18] Catherine Campbell and Carl McLean (2002) Ethnic identity, social capital and health inequalities: Factors shaping African–Caribbean participation in local community networks. *Social Science and Medicine*, 55(4), 643–657.

[19] C. Muntaner and J. Lynch (1999) Income inequality, social cohesion and class relations: A critique of Wilkinson's neo-Durkheimian research program. *International Journal of Health Services*, 29(1), 59–81.

[20] P. Gillies, K. Tolley and J. Wolstenholme (1996) Is AIDS a disease of poverty? *AIDS Care*, 8(3), 351–363.

[21] Ron Labonte (1999) Social capital and community development: Practitioner emptor. *Australia and New Zealand Journal of Public Health*, 23(4), 430–433.

[22] Ben Fine (2001) *Social capital versus social theory*. London: Routledge.

[23] Penny Hawe and Alan Shiell (2000) Social capital and health promotion: A review. *Social Science and Medicine*, 51, 871–885.

[24] Our own research in Summertown has suggested that participants in youth groups and sports clubs are less likely to be HIV-positive, but that members of *stokvels* (savings clubs, with meetings frequently associated with heavy drinking and casual partners) are significantly more likely to be HIV-positive. Catherine Campbell, Brian Williams and Denise Gilgen (2002)

Is social capital a useful conceptual tool for exploring community level influences on HIV infection? An exploratory case study from South Africa. *AIDS Care*, 14(1), 41–55.

²⁵ F. Baum, R. Bush, C. Modra, C. Murray, E. Cox, K. Alexander and R. Potter (2000) Epidemiology of participation: An Australian community study. *Journal of Epidemiology and Community Health*, 54, 414–423. Daphna Birenbaum-Carmeli (1999) Parents who get what they want: On the empowerment of the powerful. *The Sociological Review*, pp. 62–91.

²⁶ Jo Beall (1998) Social capital in waste – a solid investment? *Journal of International Development*, 9(7), 951–961.

²⁷ Most notable among these is Robert Putnam, the most famous exponent of social capital, whose neglect of the economic and political dimensions of social capital has contributed to a great deal of the bad press that the concept has received. See Fine (2001), cited above.

²⁸ Pierre Bourdieu (1986) The forms of capital. In J. Richardson (Ed) *Handbook of theory and research for the sociology of education*, pp. 241–248. New York: Greenwood.

²⁹ Hannah Arendt (1958) *The human condition*. Chicago: University of Chicago Press.

³⁰ Sandra Jovchelovitch (1996) Peripheral communities and the transformation of social representations: Queries on power and recognition. *Social Psychological Review*, 1(1), 16–26, p. 19.

³¹ Ibid.

³² Catherine Campbell and Sandra Jovchelovitch (2000) Health, community and development: Towards a social psychology of participation. *Journal of Community and Applied Social Psychology*, 10, 255–270.

³³ Ibid.

³⁴ Marshall Kreuter (1997) National level assessment of community health promotion using indicators of social capital. WHO/EURO Working Group Report. CDC, Atlanta.

³⁵ Ibid., p. 2.

³⁶ Robert Putnam (2000) *Bowling Alone: The collapse and revival of American community*. New York: Simon and Schuster.

³⁷ In this book, the concept of 'bridging social capital' includes those connections between marginalized groupings and representatives of more powerful bodies in the public and private sectors, which are sometimes referred to as 'linking social capital', e.g. by writers such as Simon Szreter (2002). The state of social capital: Bringing back in power, politics and history. *Theory and Society* (in press).

³⁸ L. Manderson and L. Whiteford (2000) *Global health policy, local realities: The fallacy of a level playing field*. Boulder: Lynne Rienner.

³⁹ Susan Saegert, J. Phillip Thompson and Mark R. Warren (2001) *Social capital in poor communities*. New York: Russell Sage Foundation.

⁴⁰ M. Barnes (1997) *Care, communities and citizens*. London: Longman.

⁴¹ Campbell and Jovchelovitch (2000), cited above.

⁴² S. Asthana and R. Oostvogels (1996) Community participation in HIV prevention. Problems and prospects for community-based strategies amongst female sex workers in Madras. *Social Science and Medicine*, 43(2), 133–148.

⁴³ 'One of the key ideological and political problems in mobilizing social capital … is not only that of empowering the very poor with the capacity to participate in bridging social capital, but, equally, of inducing the very rich and powerful to bridge much more with the rest of their fellow humans.' Szreter (2002), cited above.

## CHAPTER 4 pp. 63–82

¹ White makes a similar point in relation to sex workers in Nairobi in the mid-twentieth century, arguing that the colonial authorities turned a blind eye to their presence because the availability of commercial sex served as a force stabilizing the male migrant workforce. Luise White (1990) *The comforts of home: Prostitution in colonial Nairobi*. Chicago: Chicago University Press.

² At the time these interviews were conducted, R20 was equivalent to about £2.

³ H. Pickering, J. Todd, D. Dunn, J. Pepin and A. Wilkins (1992) Prostitutes and their clients: A Gambian survey. *Social Science and Medicine*, 34(1), 75–88.

[4] Priscilla Ulin (1992) African women and AIDS: Negotiating behavioural change. *Social Science and Medicine*, 34(1), 63–73. UN AIDS (2001c) *Gender and AIDS almanac*. Geneva: UN AIDS. Amy Kaler (2001) 'It's some kind of women's empowerment': The ambiguity of the female condom as a marker of female empowerment. *Social Science and Medicine*, 52, 783–796.

[5] Caroline Moser (1998) The asset vulnerability framework: Reassessing urban poverty reduction strategies. *World Development*, 26(1), 1–19. See also Carolyn Baylies and Janet Bujra (2000) *Aids, sexuality and gender in Africa*. London: Routledge. Ida Susser and Zena Stein (2000) Culture, sexuality and women's agency in the prevention of HIV/AIDS in South Africa. *American Journal of Public Health*, 90, 1042–1048.

[6] Nolene Dube and David Wilson (1999) Peer education programmes. In Brian Williams, Catherine Campbell and Catherine MacPhail (Eds) *Managing HIV/AIDS in South Africa: Lessons from industrial settings*. Johannesburg: CSIR. N. Ngugi, D. Wilson, J. Sebstad, F. Plummer and S. Moses (1996) Focused peer-mediated educational programmes among female sex workers to reduce sexually transmitted disease and human immunodeficiency virus transmission in Kenya and Zimbabwe. *Journal of Infectious Diseases*, 174 (suppl. 2), S240–S247.

[7] David Wilson (1995) Community peer education to prevent STD/HIV/AIDS among women in Zimbabwe and Zambia. Unpublished report by the Project Support Group, Psychology Department, University of Zimbabwe.

[8] E. Maxine Ankrah (1993) The impact of HIV/AIDS on the family and other significant relationships: The African clan revisited. *AIDS Care*, 5, 5–22.

# CHAPTER 5 pp. 83–100

[1] These interviews were conducted by the Summertown social science evaluation team, consisting of the author, colleague Catherine MacPhail, and a number of co-interviewers fluent in African languages.

[2] Jeyes fluid is an outdoor disinfectant containing tar acids, more commonly used for cleaning drains.

[3] Peer educators received this money as an honorarium, in exchange for their commitment to devote two hours a day to their peer-educational activities.

[4] Chapters 10 and 11 will outline the obstacles that stood in the way of the Project's attempts to implement peer education among mineworkers.

[5] Fran Baum (1999b) The role of social capital in health promotion: Australian perspectives. *Health Promotion Journal of Australia*, 9(3), 171–178. A. Portes and P. Landolt (1996) The downside of social capital. *The American Prospect*, 26, 18–21.

# CHAPTER 6 pp. 101–118

[1] Mkhondzeni Gumede (2001) Panel discussant at the AIDS in Context conference, University of the Witwatersrand, April 2001.

[2] Paulo Freire (1973/1993b) *Education for critical consciousness*. New York: Continuum.

[3] Hélène Joffe (1999) *Risk and 'the other'*. Cambridge: Cambridge University Press.

[4] B. Thom, M. Kelly, S. Harris and A. Holling (1999) *Alcohol: Measuring the impact of community initiatives*. London: Health Education Authority.

[5] UN AIDS (2001) *Gender and AIDS Almanac*. Geneva: UN AIDS.

[6] Mark Warren, J. Phillip Thompson and Susan Saegert (2001) The role of social capital in combating poverty. In Susan Saegert, J. Phillip Thompson and Mark R. Warren (Eds) (2001) *Social capital and poor communities*. New York: Russell Sage Foundation.

[7] Michael Woolcock (1998) Social capital and economic development: Towards a theoretical synthesis and policy framework. *Theory and Society*, 27, 151–208.

[8] Naila Kabeer (1994) *Reversed realities: Gender hierarchies in development thought*. New Delhi: Kali for Women.

# CHAPTER 7 pp. 121–131

[1] In South Africa, the term 'learner' is favoured over 'pupil' or 'scholar'.

[2] Brian Williams, Denise Gilgen, Catherine Campbell, Dirk Taljaard and Catherine MacPhail (2000) *The natural history of HIV/AIDS in South Africa: A biomedical and social survey.* Johannesburg: CSIR.

[3] Dennis J. Dobbs (2000) *Summertown: South Africa. Results of the Second Community-based Survey.* Report to US Population Council, New York.

[4] These issues are reviewed in Catherine MacPhail, Brian Williams and Catherine Campbell (2002) Relative risk of HIV infection amongst young men and women in a South African township. *International Journal of STIs and AIDS*, 13(5), 331–342.

[5] Ibid. Also S. Gregson, C. Nyamukapa and others (in press) Sexual mixing patterns and sex-differentials in teenage exposure to HIV infection in rural Zimbabwe. *The Lancet.*

[6] According to MacPhail, Williams and Campbell (cited above), 25% of Summertown women aged between 15 and 25 who had only had one sexual partner were HIV-positive.

[7] Brian Williams et al. (2000), cited above.

[8] Quotations in this section come from focus groups. Separate focus groups were conducted for men and women, divided according to 13–16, 17–20 and 21–25-year age groups.

[9] Catherine Campbell (1995) The social identity of township youth (parts 1 and 2). *South African Journal of Psychology*, 25(3), 150–167.

[10] S. Abdool Karim, Q. Abdool Karim, E. Preston-Whyte and N. Sankar (1992) Reasons for lack of condom use among high school students. *South African Medical Journal*, 82, 107–110. A. Akande (1997) Black South African adolescents' attitudes towards AIDS precautions. *School Psychology International*, 18, 325–341.

[11] Deepa Narayan (2000) *Can anybody hear us? (Voices of the poor)* New York: Oxford University Press.

[12] R. Jewkes, N. Abrahams and Z. Mvo (1998) Why do nurses abuse patients? Reflections from South African obstetric services. *Social Science and Medicine*, 47(11).

[13] Simon Gregson, Heather Waddell and Stephen Chandiwana (2001) School education and HIV control in sub-Saharan Africa: From discord to harmony? *Journal of International Development*, 13, 467–485.

[14] Josina Machel (2001) Unsafe sexual behaviour amongst schoolgirls in Mocambique: A matter of gender and class. *Reproductive Health Matters*, 9(17), 82–92.

[15] Joseph Collins (2000) *Aids in the context of development.* UN RISD, Paper 4, December.

[16] C. Varga and L. Mkubalo (1996) Sexual (non)negotiation among black African teenagers in Durban. *Agenda*, 28, 31–38. K. Wood and R. Jewkes (1997) Violence, rape and sexual coercion: Everyday love in a South African township. *Gender and Development*, 5, 41–46. K. Wood, F. Maforah and R. Jewkes (1998) 'He forced me to love him': Putting violence on adolescent sexual health agendas. *Social Science and Medicine*, 47, 233–242.

[17] Lisa Vetten and Kailash Bhana (2001) *Violence, vengeance and gender. A preliminary investigation into the links between violence against women and HIV/AIDS in South Africa.* Johannesburg: Centre for the Study of Violence and Reconciliation.

# CHAPTER 8 pp. 132–148

[1] P. Christie and C. Collins (1982). Bantu education: Apartheid ideology or labour reproduction. *Comparative Education*, 18(1), 59–75.

[2] Review Committee on Curriculum 2005 (2000). *A South African Curriculum for the Twenty-first Century.* Pretoria: Report of the Review Committee on Curriculum 2005 to Minister of Education, Kadar Asmal, 31 May 2000.

[3] M. Cross (1993). Youths, culture and politics in South African education: The past, present, and future. *Youth and Society*, 24(4), 377–398.

[4] Campbell and Jovchelovich (2000), cited above.

[5] Peter Aggleton and Catherine Campbell (2000) Working with young people: Towards an agenda for sexual health policy. *Sex and Relationship Therapy*, 15(3), 283–296.

[6] Ibid.

[7] Ibid.

[8] Robert Putnam (1993) *Making democracy work*. Princeton: Princeton University Press. Robert Putnam (2000) *Bowling Alone: The collapse and revival of American community*. New York: Simon and Schuster.

[9] Brian Williams, Catherine MacPhail, Catherine Campbell, Dirk Taljaard, Eleanor Gouws, Solly Moema, Zodwa Mzaidume and Bareng Rasego (2000) The Summertown Project: Limiting transmission of HIV through community participation. *South African Journal of Science*, 96(6), 351–359.

[10] Virginia Morrow (2001) *Networks and neighborhoods: Children's and young people's perspectives*. London: Health Development Agency.

## CHAPTER 9 pp. 151–165

[1] Catherine Campbell and Brian Williams (1999) Understanding the impact of a community-led HIV prevention programme: Context, conceptual framework and methodology. *Australian Journal of Primary Health*, 15(4), 9–23.

[2] Brian Williams, Bertran Auvert, Dirk Taljaard and others (2002) The response of a South African mining community to the epidemic of HIV in the context of a major intervention programme. Draft paper, 31 March 2002. Brian Williams and others (forthcoming) Changing patterns of knowledge, reported behaviour and sexually transmitted infections in a South African gold mining community. *AIDS*.

[3] For various reasons people may tell survey researchers that they have been using condoms, even if this is not the case.

[4] David Ginsburg (2000) Report to the stakeholders in the Summertown Project. Unpublished report to the Summertown Project Stakeholder Committee.

[5] Brian Williams and Eleanor Gouws (2001) Partial comparison of the 1998 and 2000 Summertown surveys. Unpublished discussion document.

[6] Jonathan Crush, Theresa Ulicki, Teke Tseane and Elizabeth Jansen van Vuuren (2001) Undermining labour: The rise of sub-contracting in South African gold mines. *Journal of Southern African Studies*, 27(1), 5–31.

[7] Peter Evans (1996) Government action, social capital and development: Reviewing the evidence on synergy. *World Development*, 24(6), 1119–1132. Patrick Heller (1996) Social capital as a product of class mobilization and state intervention: Industrial workers in Kerala, India. *World Development*, 24(6), 1055–1071.

[8] Helen Schneider and Joanne Stein (2000) Implementing AIDS policy in post-apartheid South Africa. *Social Science and Medicine*, 52, 723–731.

[9] South African scientists deplore their government's meddling. *The Economist*, 6 April 2002, p. 85.

[10] Lisa Vetten and Kailash Bhana (2001) *Violence, vengeance and gender. A preliminary investigation into the links between violence against women and HIV/AIDS in South Africa*. Johannesburg: Centre for the Study of Violence and Reconciliation.

[11] State fury over AZT for raped baby. *Mail and Guardian*, 11–17 January 2002.

[12] Salim Abdool Karrim and 21 others (2002) Vertical HIV transmission in South Africa: Translating research into policy and practice. *Lancet*, 359 (9311), 992.

[13] At the time of writing there is some welcome evidence that the government is starting to relax its hard-line anti-drugs position. AIDS activists welcome this as the potential start of a new and more positive role for South African leaders in relation to the epidemic. Government stages a dramatic about-turn on its AIDS policy. *Business Day*, 18 April 2002.

[14] Roy Williams (1998) *Project report: Stakeholder Evaluation. Summertown HIV/STD Intervention Project*. University of Reading: Education for Development, p. 28.

[15] A. Trapido, N. Mqoqi, C. Macheke, A. Davies and C. Panter (1996) Occupational lung disease in ex-mineworkers – sound a further alarm. *South African Medical Journal*, 86(5), 559. A. Trapido, N. Mqoqi, B. Williams, N. White, A. Solomon, R. Goode, C. Macheke, A. Davies and C. Panter (1998) Prevalence of occupational lung disease in a random sample of former mineworkers, Libode District, Eastern Cape Province, South Africa. *American Journal of Industrial Medicine*, 34, 305–311.

[16] E. Corbett, G. Churchyard, T. Clayton, P. Herselman, B. Williams, R. Hayes, D. Mulder and K. de Cock (1999) Risk factors for pulmonary mycobacterial disease in South African miners. *American Journal of Critical Care Medicine*, 159, 94–99.


# CHAPTER 10 pp. 166–182

[1] Catherine MacPhail, Catherine Campbell and Marian Pitts (submitted for publication) 'Who can cure AIDS?' The role of traditional healers in diagnosing and treating STIs and HIV/AIDS.

[2] Eventually, after much mediation and intervention by peacemaking individuals, a compromise was reached whereby the selection committee for interviewers consisted of equal numbers of academics and non-academics (grassroots people), and the survey went ahead.

[3] STI results were never linked to people's names, but only to anonymous numbered cards, which local people presented in order to get their results. HIV results were not given to people, but survey participants who wanted their HIV results were referred to a clinic where they could be tested and counselled at no cost.

[4] I am grateful to Teddy Brett for helpful discussions of this point. See also E.A. Brett (1997) Participation and accountability in development administration. Unpublished discussion document, Development Studies Institute, LSE.


# CONCLUSION pp. 183–196

[1] UN AIDS (2000) *Report on the global HIV/AIDS epidemic*. Geneva: UN AIDS.

[2] The concept of 'political will' has been criticized as vague and imprecise by some who argue that lack of appropriate action in response to the HIV epidemic is the result of 'political choices', made very consciously and deliberately by powerful social actors, rather than the result of mysterious collective social processes.

[3] E.g. UN AIDS (2000), cited above; UN AIDS (2002) *Report on the global HIV/AIDS epidemic: 2002*. Geneva: UN AIDS.

[4] Pierre Bourdieu (1985) The forms of capital. In John Richardson (Ed) *Handbook of theory and research for the sociology of education*. New York: Greenwood.

[5] Hélène Joffe (1999) *Risk and 'the other'*. Cambridge: Cambridge University Press. R. Crawford (1994) The boundaries of self and the unhealthy other: Reflections on health, culture and AIDS. *Social Science and Medicine*, 38(10) 1347–1365.

[6] Tony Barnett and Alan Whiteside (2002) *AIDS in the 21st century: Disease and globalization*. New York: Palgrave Macmillan. See Farmer (1992) for a discussion of the international context of the HIV/AIDS epidemic in Haiti. Paul Farmer (1992) *Aids and accusation: Haiti and the geography of blame*. Berkeley: University of California Press.

[7] L. Botes and D. van Rensburg (2000) Community participation in development: Nine plagues and twelve commandments. *Community Development Journal*, 35(1), 41–58.

[8] Ruairi Brugha and Gill Walt (2001) A global health fund: A leap of faith? *British Medical Journal*, 323, 152–154, July.

[9] Fiona Fleck (2002) Global Fund overwhelmed by requests. *British Medical Journal*, 324, 807.

[10] Peter Piot (2000) Global AIDS epidemic: time to turn the tide. *Science*, 299, 2176–2178.

[11] Ruairi Brugha, Mary Starling and Gill Walt (2002) GAVI, the first steps: Lessons for the Global Fund. *Lancet*, 359, 435–438.

CPSIA information can be obtained at www.ICGtesting.com
Printed in the USA
LVOW060209210112

264937LV00001B/3/P